Positive Parenting
Fitness A Total Approach to Caring for the Physical and Emotional Needs of Your New Family

Positive Parenting
Fitness
A Total Approach to Caring for the Physical and Emotional Needs of Your New Family

Sylvia Klein Olkin, MS

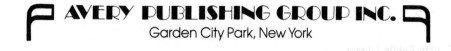
AVERY PUBLISHING GROUP INC.
Garden City Park, New York

The medical and health procedures in this book are based on the training, personal experiences, and research of the author. Because each person and situation is unique, the editor and the publisher urge the reader to check with a qualified health professional before using any procedure where there is any question as to its appropriateness.

The publisher does not advocate the use of any particular diet or exercise program but believes the information presented in this book should be available to the public.

Because there is always some risk involved, the author and publisher are not responsible for any adverse effects or consequences resulting from the use of any of the suggestions, preparations, or procedures in this book. Please do not use the book if you are unwilling to assume the risk. Feel free to consult a physician or other qualified health professional. It is a sign of wisdom, not cowardice, to seek a second or third opinion.

Cover Design: Rudy Shur and Janine Eisner-Wall
Cover Art: Janine Eisner-Wall
In-House Editor: Marie Caratozzolo
Typesetter: Widget Design, Mount Marion, NY

Technical Advisor: Carl Mailhot, BS, PT

Library of Congress Cataloging-in-Publication Data

Olkin, Sylvia Klein.
    Positive parenting fitness : a parent's resource guide to
    nutrition, stress reduction, total exercise, and practical
    information / Sylvia Klein Olkin.
        p. cm.
    Includes index.
    ISBN 0-89529-481-8
    1. Postnatal care. 2. Exercise for women. 3. Physical fitness.
    I. Title.
    RG801.045 1992
    613.7'045—dc20   91-28933
                                                            CIP

Printed in the United States of America

10 9 8 7 6 5 4 3 2 1

Contents

This book is dedicated with love to my grandmother
Rose Farstendiger Statman (1898-1956).
She gave me unconditional love, saved my life on numerous occasions,
took me out for "secret" Chinese-food lunches,
taught me how to bake, and also how to challenge life.
In the thirteen short years we had together,
she taught by example about loving and parenting.
Those lessons that she taught me,
I have the privilege to share with you through this book.

Acknowledgments

For the last eight years, very many generous and devoted individuals supported and nurtured me as I worked on the realization of this book. The creation, development, and finally the completion of it would not have been possible without the considerate efforts of a special group of caring people. My heartfelt thanks to:

Bob Olkin, my husband of twenty-six years, who on August 30, 1989, rushed me to the hospital and literally saved my life. (I had pneumonia and couldn't breathe.) Your constant love and concern enabled me to complete this book.

Mat and Mike Olkin, my sons, who are always there with an easy joke and an optimistic way of living and loving life. Thanks for enabling me to discover the joys and frustrations of being a parent.

Meyer and Nora Klein, my parents, for your dependable care and concern in so many untold ways.

Helaine Ronen, my sister, who, with humor and affection, contributes enormously to my healing.

Sylvia Olkin, my mother-in-law, for being the best mother-in-law a woman can have.

My huge, loving family, especially aunts Mollie Seletsky, Florence Sakow, and Eleanor Osofsky; my sisters-in-law Arlene Olkin and Jewel McGarry, who called, sent innumerable "get well" cards, and visited throughout my various bouts in and out of the hospital.

Nancy and Paul Cohen, steadfast friends through the fun times and the sad moments.

My neurologists, David Shiling, MD, Anthony Alessi, MD, and Anis Racy, MD, who have treated me with genuine caring and fondness throughout the rough times.

Bonni Piccione, my loyal part-time secretary, for proofreading and critiquing much of this book.

Jill Wasserman, new mother, for your helpful suggestions and support.

Bonnie Allyn, new mother, for strength and love when I was at my worst.

Bonnie, Robbie, Todd, John, and Suzanne Tomlinson, my Vermont family, for showing me what good family life really means.

Naomi and David Howe, dear friends, who posed — so long ago — for the massage photographs in a freezing studio!

Elizabeth Noble, PT, for sharing your concerns and dreams about postpartum fitness.

Dr. Guss, my children's pediatrician par excellence, and his lovely wife for continued support and encouragement.

Maureen Braun, RN, BN, Positive Pregnancy/Parenting Master Teacher, director of Bodies and Babies (a pre- and postpartum fitness program in Bellingham, WA), and a delightful friend and artist. With your drawings, you have helped this book come alive with vitality, clarity, and joyfulness. Thanks especially for all of your editorial advice and help in the creation of Chapter Fourteen, "Exercises Designed to Relieve Backaches."

Lois Rivard, a reliable, committed friend and artist, for creating the line drawings for the acupressure chapter and various other illustrations.

Antonia, for your illustration Sleep When the Baby Sleeps in Chapter Four.

Sandy Lucas, for your herb drawings.

Jacquie Burzycki, RN, Positive Parenting Fitness Master Teacher, and Paige Rushford for posing for the photos on which many of the illustrations in this book are based. Thanks especially for your help on the guidelines for the aerobic exercises and the nutrition chapter, and for being dear friends.

Carl Mailhot, BS, PT, whose technical expertise and judgment have added so much to this book.

Carroll Mailhot, Positive Parenting Fitness certified teacher, for the walks and talks we shared during the creation of this book.

Diane Milhan, PhD, PT, Positive Parenting Fitness instructor, for volunteering to share your technical knowledge in the creation of the practice guidelines and aerobic chapter.

Liz Schneider, BFA, Positive Parenting Fitness instructor, dancer and choreographic consultant, for creating and writing the Mother/Baby Exercises and for the practice video of routines.

Mary Beth Murray, MS, and Alayne C. Salvador, BA, certified aerobic and Positive Parenting Fitness instructors, for patiently designing, photographing, and revising all of the strength-training and low-impact aerobic exercises. Thanks to your technical skill and knowledge, postpartum women will shape up!

Ann Cowlin, MA, director of Dancing Thru Pregnancy, pre- and postpartum fitness programs, Branford, CT, for your creation of Constructive Relaxation (Chapter Two) and for being the kind of friend who readily shares her expertise. We will get the Perinatal Health and Fitness Network off the ground. . . .

Pamela Shrock, PhD, for your expertise in Chapter Seven, for writing an outstanding preface, and for your caring and support along the way. Just knowing you is a blessing!

Liz Fracchia, RN, Positive Pregnancy Fitness Master Teacher, and a first-rate friend. Thanks for all of your expertise in the nursing chapter.

Terry Mooney, RN, International Certified Lactation Consultant (IBCLC), for your useful suggestions regarding nursing.

Paula Mara Lyons, OT, the very first Positive Pregnancy Fitness trained instructor, for sending the article on postpartum depression.

Linda Green, RN, DPA, for your helpful contributions to the chapter on natural remedies.

Dr. Richard Geller and Marcy Geller for your help in the creation of the baby movement chapter.

Susun Weed, author and herbalist, and Jeannine Parvati Baker, yoga teacher, author, and herbalist, for expert advice in Chapter Three, "Remedies for Common Ailments of New Mothers."

Miriam Erick, RD, of Brigham and Women's Hospital, Boston, MA, Nutrition Department, for your expertise and menus in the chapter on nutrition.

Penny Simkin, PT, for your supportive counsel and good advice.

Vimala Schneider McClure, director of the International Association of Infant Massage Instructors, and Rebecca Goldstein, Certified Infant Massage Specialist, for invaluable contributions to the baby massage chapter.

Grace Burkhardt, RN, acupressure specialist, for researching and helping in the creation of the acupressure section.

Tina Gavlick for your expert advice on peer counseling and for your accessibility.

Carl Jones, CCE, author of numerous childbirth education books and dedicated friend, who wrote numerous hilarious letters to me while I was in the hospital, and who gave me many ideas for the blues chapter.

Geri Flynn, RN, Certified Positive Pregnancy/Parenting Fitness Master Teacher, for your moral support, expertise, and ready smile.

Lynn Moen, director of the Birth and Life Bookstore, Seattle, WA, for your superb help in preparing this book's detailed bibliography. Special thanks for always being gracious and supportive.

JoAnn Agnello, Positive Pregnancy/Parenting Fitness Master Teacher, Registered Therapeutic Massage Therapist, for helping to prepare the massage bibliography.

Rudy Shur, managing editor at Avery, who, as usual, waited a long, long time for the birth of this book. It was a very difficult pregnancy, labor, and delivery, but you had prodigious patience balanced with genuine caring.

Marie Caratozzolo, my editor at Avery, for your creative, organizational, and exacting suggestions during the editing process. You and co-editor Linda Comac made me work very hard and demanded the best from me, and this book is better for it.

The over 650 trained Positive Pregnancy and Parenting Fitness instructors across the country, in Canada, and in England who wanted a text on parenting fitness. *Well, here it is!* Thanks to your commitment, encouragement, suggestions, and ideas, Positive Pregnancy and Positive Parenting Fitness is growing and prospering.

All the new mothers, fathers, and babies of the world. I wish you faith, joy, and peace.

Sylvia Klein Olkin

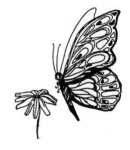

Preface

Pregnancy is that special state that conjures up the promise of the future for expectant parents. It is a time of hopes, dreams, and the anticipation of this new creation, this fetus, whose perceptible movements in utero, benign hiccup or pressure on the mother's spine, give credence to its very existence. During what seems, for most, to be an interminably long nine months, many parents-to-be give full vent to their fantasies, imagining their new life as a family, wondering what life will be like with a child, and what kind of parents they will be.

For some, pregnancy is experienced as a major life event for which much forethought is needed to cope with the added responsibility. Concrete plans must be made for accommodating the new baby. There may be possible changes in a career, the need to reshuffle finances or work schedules, or to arrange for baby care. Some parents-to-be see the pregnancy as a "rite of passage" as they move from one life stage to the next; some see it as a prelude to fulfillment of themselves as men or women in their new roles as parents.

The postpartum period can be exciting, thrilling, exhilarating, and novel. It is also a time of immense challenge: a time of vulnerability fraught with difficulties as the couple attempts to balance the life that *was* with the reality of the life that *is.* Husband and wife may need to cast aside unrealistic expectations of maintaining their former lifestyle and learn to forego their own personal needs, wants, and desires as a couple. No matter how well they might have planned, they are often astounded at how much of their time, attention, and energy is needed to devote to their baby, whose incessant demands are borne from its helplessness and utter dependence on its parents.

Parents-to-be have few opportunities to prepare for the arduous task of parenting and child rearing. It is not, therefore, surprising that so many new parents feel inadequate for the responsibilities and pressures that accompany their bundle of joy. In fact, many feel overwhelmed by the enormity of the tasks demanded, combined with the need to maintain some time and energy for themselves and their relationship.

How can one become "fit to parent"? For over thirty years, there has been a proliferation of classes regarding childbirth preparation and education: classes designed to enable expectant women and couples to become active participants in the events surrounding the birth of their child. Along with pregnancy fitness programs, the knowledge, skills, and an understanding of the emotional aspects of the birthing process have enabled couples to share the powerful physical and emotional work necessary for the birth.

Preparation for actual parenting and for the vicissitudes of the postpartum period have been, in general, sadly neglected. Hospitals and perinatal instructors seldom organize classes to prepare couples for these events; in fact, they have been accused in the past of "leaving the new parents on the delivery table."

Books, though few in number, tend to focus on the needs of the newborn and to give advice on the "how-to's" of baby care. Few manuals give sorely needed directives for "couple care" or "mother care" or "father care," which would enable new parents to feel "fit to parent." Sylvia Klein Olkin has written a much-needed book that provides answers to the many questions new parents have: questions about the social and physical changes in their lives, and about the emotional stays that hold their relationship together. This book provides the answers that will enable couples to fulfill their new roles as parents.

Sylvia Olkin's book is characterized by a holistic approach to the "fitness of parenting." There is an underlying belief that a positive attitude toward parenting and that being "fit to parent" depend also on "fitness" of body and soul. To provide for the well-being of both body and mind, the book presents proper nutrition, rest and relaxation skills, physical rehabilitation through stretching and breathing exercises, activities to revitalize Mom and Dad's relationship, and mother-baby exercises for fun and interaction. Sylvia Klein Olkin's material is drawn from down-to-earth information and natural, simple, homey advice, stemming from good old common sense and centuries-old wisdom.

An experienced self-development teacher and childbirth educator, Sylvia Klein Olkin knows of what she speaks and writes. She brings to her book a strongly subjective approach. This subjectivity, however, is born out of years of working closely with and gaining feedback from the perinatal woman and her partner during the physical and emotional experiences of pregnancy and postpartum. For years, she has conducted training programs for professionals in the field of childbirth education, obstetrical nursing, and exercise therapy. She has constantly added new dimensions that are bound to help perinatal women and couples. Her knowledge has constantly been reconfirmed through a wealth of learning, updating, teaching, and applying of her skills and information with dedication and practicality.

From all of her rich and varied life experiences—including her own parenting—Sylvia Klein Olkin has given her text an authenticity that her readers, both lay and professional, will sense and find extremely helpful as they live through or teach about the ebb and flow of the parenting years.

Pamela Shrock, PhD, ACCE
Director of Psycho-Somatic OB/GYN
Winthrop University Hospital
Mineola, New York

PART I
Welcome to Parenthood

CHAPTER ONE

Positive Parenting Fitness: An Overview

Congratulations! A new role and a new person have just been added to your life. You are experiencing many new and often challenging situations because of these changes. You may not think of being a parent as playing a new role, but this description has helped many of my Positive Parenting Fitness students to have a new and clearer perspective of their lives. Many new parents get so seriously involved with the responsibility of being a parent, they forget that the role has some very enjoyable and humorous aspects. It may take a while for you to develop some confidence in yourself and your abilities as a parent. Once you have had some time and practice to get more familiar with the role and its possibilities, you can learn to be successful as a parent and to enjoy it at the same time.

Positive Parenting Fitness offers a four-step approach to physical fitness and positive thinking for mental stability and enjoyment of your life as a new parent. Whenever you assume a new role in your life, such as being a teacher, an engineer, an artist, or a parent, it is beneficial to have some guidelines to help you succeed in that role. Positive Parenting Fitness contains helpful guidelines based on ancient wisdom combined with the latest knowledge for new and busy parents.

ANCIENT WISDOM AND MODERN ADVICE

The collective wisdom from past generations of new parents is invaluable for today's new parents. These "tricks of the trade" or simple remedies for current situations can help you over the first sleepless weeks with your new infant. Since we don't live in extended families anymore, much of the wisdom that was usually passed from mother to daughter to baby is being lost. The Positive Parenting Fitness program combines natural, effective advice and wisdom with current research. All of the practical, easy-to-use advice and support in this program is designed for you and your baby.

A BALANCED, HARMONIOUS, PHYSICAL AND MENTAL APPROACH

New parents often find stability and harmony are lost as soon as the new baby enters their lives. Routines are disrupted because of the new baby's needs. Due to lack of sleep and frustrations with the new baby, a new mother may feel disheartened. A new father might adjust to his new role well but may still crave the way things used to be. New parenting is a rocky and transitional period in life. The Positive Parenting Fitness program was developed to be an important support for new parents during this pivotal point in their lives.

This book has been divided into three main parts. Part I deals with common areas of new parenting that cause the most concern. This unique time undoubtedly causes changes, both physical and mental, that should be addressed.

"Stress Management for New Parents" is a chapter that presents a potpourri of approaches to strengthen your mental state during those first trying weeks of parenthood. Sometimes, just breathing slowly and deliberately will calm you down during stressful moments. Other times, you may need to get away from your baby for a while. Living with a new baby is a "here and now" experience: you never know what the next moment will bring.

The importance of a healthy and balanced postpartum diet is addressed in "Postpartum Nutrition." Properly nourishing your postpartum body can ease the nursing mother's worries of adequately feeding her infant. Included is a safe weight-reduction program with recipes that are especially nutritious for nursing mothers. As breastfeeding mothers are responsible for adequately feeding their new babies, detailed information on proper nutrition is presented for a healthy body and baby.

"Understanding and Coping with the 'Blues'" is designed to give you a better understanding of situations that might get you down and offers suggestions on what you can do to alleviate them. The sensible advice to *sleep when your baby sleeps* has helped thousands of mothers.

The chapter "Remedies for Common Ailments of New Mothers" can help ease your worries and put you into a better frame of mind. The holistic approach found in this area combines both physical and mental techniques to ease your stress and increase your enjoyment during the early days of new parenting. The wisdom of past generations of women on the use of herbs for healing, combined with modern scientific information on the healing process, will help ease your first months postpartum.

"Reawakening Your Sexual Self" explains why some new mothers have problems adjusting to a sexual life after the birth of a baby and describes how to remedy that situation. Also featured is a thorough discussion on birth control methods so you can avoid getting pregnant again sooner than you want.

The actual Positive Parenting Fitness exercise program is found in Part II. This four-step program, which was developed based on ten years of Positive Parenting Fitness classes, will surely satisfy all your physical needs. The physical regimen begins right after delivery; it starts with healing, stretching, and breathing exercises. The program naturally progresses to low-impact aerobics and concludes with shaping-up exercises designed to tone those common postpartum trouble spots. Also included are strength-training exercises (for "kid carrying").

Part III focuses on exercising as a family unit. It includes a delightful mother/baby workout, a unique exercise series for dads and babies, and some exercises that can be done as a family. Also included are specific exercises that can be done with your baby as a natural part of your daily routine. Two special chapters, "Baby Massage and Acupressure" and "Baby Movement Program," encourage you to spend special time stimulating and stretching your new little one. What a pleasurable experience awaits you!

HOW OUR BRAINS FUNCTION

Some new mothers complain that their brains have stopped functioning since their baby arrived. With inadequate sleep and taking care of the baby night and day, you may feel the same way. But you may not have realized that stability and peace are achieved by balancing our rational selves with our intuitive selves. Our tendency is to overwork the rational, outer-directed, programmed part of the brain, while simply ignoring the inner-directed, intuitive, creative side. Learning how to build pathways between the two halves of your brain will increase your potential and total enjoyment of life. When dealing with your new baby, you will have to rely on your intuition and feelings about certain situations because your baby will not learn to talk for a very long time. Figure 1.1 is a representation of the Split Brain Theory, which explains the different functions served by the left and right hemispheres of the brain. You will notice that the brain's left side is thought to control our rational and outer-directed selves. This side deals with such processes as linear thinking, verbal and routine memory, logical thought, mechanical and analytical thinking, and the actions that go along with our thoughts. The right side is thought to control our irrational and inner-directed selves. This side of the brain deals with intuition, our artistic and creative selves, spatial relations, meditative spaces, visual images, and aesthetics. Getting these two very different parts of ourselves to work together in harmony is what the Positive Parenting Fitness program is all about.

Since we are a society that is based largely on scientific research, is it any wonder that we tend to ignore the right side of the brain? We are constantly doing things, studying things, and analyzing things. In addition, we like to believe that everything in our lives is rational and logical. So we tend to ignore any sinking feeling that warns of danger to ourselves and our babies.

With a new baby in your life, you will notice the need to rely on your intuition more often. If you sense that there is something wrong with your child, you may not have a logical explanation, but you may have to "go with" your feelings. The Positive Parenting Fitness program encourages you to believe in yourself and in your capacities as a new parent. You will learn that fine tuning your senses and your intuition will help you more than most of the parenting books written by the "experts." Our parenting program encourages you to tune into your body and your baby in order to make parenting a more enjoyable and less stressful experience.

Figure 1.1   The Split Brain

Left Brain* (Right Side of Body)		**Right Brain** (Left Side of Body)
Rational Outer-directed		Irrational Inner-directed
Speech/Verbal Programmed Logical/Mathematical Linear/Detailed Controlled Intellectual Dominant Active Analytic Reading/Writing/Naming Sequential Ordering		Spatial/Musical Holistic Artistic/Symbolic Simultaneous Emotional Intuitive/Creative Spiritual/Oneness Receptive Visual Acceptance Infinite Feeling
Complex Order Complex Motor Sequences		Perceptions of Abstract Patterns Recognition of Abstract Figures

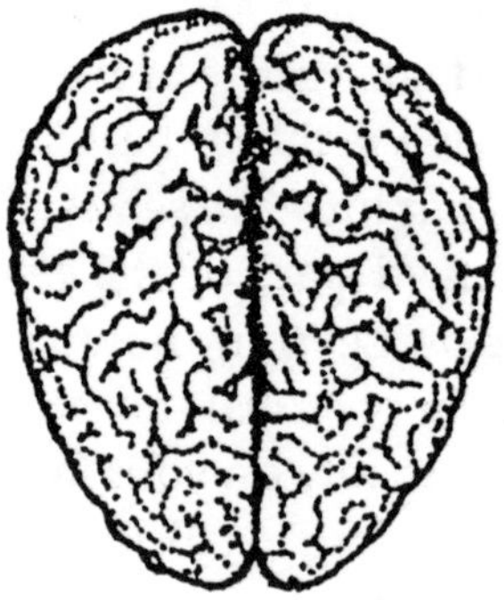

*Note that in a few people the functions are reversed.

FAITH AND DISCIPLINE

Faith can be applied in many ways: faith in yourself and in your own abilities and talents, faith that the situation in which you find yourself is the perfect one for you, and faith that you will get help when you need it. Putting all things in their proper perspectives, the parental role requires a tremendous amount of faith. There will undoubtedly be times when your baby will cry and you will never be able to figure out why. Other times, you may find it hard to cope with your new circumstance. Often this inability to cope may be due to inadequate sleep, trying to accomplish too much in too short a time, annoying in-laws, or simple unfamiliarity with your new role. It is at these times that faith, deep breathing, and being able to laugh at yourself and your problems can be the most helpful remedies. Faith in your ability to assume the parental role will give you great leverage. You will find that you can learn not to take yourself and your new role so seriously; it is then that you will genuinely begin to enjoy it.

By incorporating stretching and breathing exercises, low-impact aerobics, strength training, mother/baby routines, and proper postpartum nutrition, you will find that you will begin to feel better physically as well as mentally; this will result in your having more energy to put into your role. The Positive Parenting Fitness program is not a cure-all; it will not change your life's situation. Think of this system, however, as a very useful set of tools that can fine tune your body and mind so you can function more efficiently in this time of increased responsibilities and duties. As you begin to include some of the program's practices in your life, you will begin to see things and situations differently. This will lead to a fuller appreciation of your new role (dirty diapers, 3 a.m. feedings, and all), and you will notice how this new role is contributing to your experience of life. Parenthood can offer you a whole new realm of experiences. By playing your new role to the fullest and calling upon all of your untapped natural talents, you will get the most enjoyment out of being a parent.

CHAPTER TWO

Stress Management for New Parents

Stress seems to be the malady of the nineties. Somehow, the pace of life these days is perpetually on fast forward. Many new parents want to (or have to) accomplish too much in too little time. Of the countless number of working mothers, many have only limited time off from their jobs, and most companies do not offer paternity leaves for new fathers. Adjusting to all the physical and emotional changes that a baby brings can be intensely stressful. This chapter suggests a multifaceted or holistic approach for managing and reducing stress. You can pick and choose those techniques that work best for you.

WHAT IS STRESS?

Stress is the way your body responds to the physical and psychological events that you experience. These responses include the physical and emotional events in your life, what you believe is happening to you now, and what you think about or worry about happening in the future.

Stress is not always a negative thing, though. There are some very positive aspects of stress that can actually make certain experiences more enjoyable. For example, stress can cause that extra burst of effort during participation in an aerobic activity or in a sports event; it can be the reason for a good physical response during lovemaking; it can be the cause of a more excited reaction while watching an athletic event or when hearing good news.

The negative aspects of stress include daily frustrations and anxieties; feelings of helplessness, of not being appreciated, and of insecurity. Stress can cause tension headaches, body aches due to tight muscles, and high blood pressure.

Learning to recognize and deal with the ways your body reacts to stress is an acquired skill. It takes time and effort as well as desire, but you can do it. The Positive Parenting Fitness program presents a multi-faceted approach to exercise and stress reduction. The program will help you comfortably follow a set of guidelines that will eventually lead you to your center of strength.

COMMON STRESSORS OF NEW PARENTS

Time Management

When a new baby enters your life, your stress level automatically goes up. Suddenly you realize that you and your partner are responsible for the baby twenty-four hours a day, seven days a week, for the next twenty-odd years. You have a new time schedule—the baby's! Even though you wanted to have this baby, you suddenly realize that you are not in control of your own time. You may feel robbed of your prepregnancy freedoms and responsibility-free life. To compound the frustration, you may feel very guilty about having these feelings. During the first few weeks of early parenthood, you may feel completely unsure of yourself because you are playing a new role.

This is a time to realistically look at your life and set new priorities for yourself. Table 2.1 presents a chart for new mothers entitled *How Am I Coping?* Filling out this chart may help you in evaluating your "new" life and in establishing your new priorities. Be aware that as your baby grows, your priorities will change. So, it might be a good idea to get out your list once every three months and rethink your priorities.

Advice . . . Advice . . . and More Advice . . .

When you have a baby, everybody seems to turn into an expert on the subject of babies. You get advice from everyone, especially your parents and your in-laws. These older-generation people in your life may have trouble adjusting to their new roles as grandmother or grandfather, yet they have endless advice on how their grandchild should be fed, changed, played with, and loved. These people who are so important in your life are well-meaning, but often they are basing their advice on what they *think* they did twenty or so years ago. Infant care has changed drastically over the last twenty years.

My Positive Pregnancy Fitness students complained endlessly about this aspect of their lives. We decided that the wisest thing to do is nod your head "yes!" and agree with all of this well-meant advice, but then do what you feel is best for your baby. After all, you are the one who spends twenty-four hours a day with your child, and you know him better than anyone else does. Believe in yourself, your own intuitions, and your parenting role.

Table 2.1   How Am I Coping?

Directions:

1. Under the Coping column, rank yourself in each area from 1 to 10, with 10 representing a high level of satisfaction and 1 representing a low level.
2. Mark "$" for those areas that cost money; mark "$$" for lots of money.
3. Mark "T" for those areas that require a lot of time; mark "t" for a little time.
4. Under the Rank column, list your top five areas of concern. Use 1 as the most important and 5 as the least important.

Area	Coping	$	Time	Rank	Intended Date for Beginning Change
1. An exercise program	*unreadable*				
2. Weight					
3. Time with baby					
4. Balance between work and leisure					
5. Nutritional diet					
6. Getting enough sleep					
7. Time alone					
8. Getting my "touch needs" met (not sex)					
9. Maintaining friendships					
10. Laughter and joy					
11. Goals for living					
12. Other					

Returning to Work

New motherhood can be especially difficult for an active career woman. Many career women in my Positive Parenting Fitness classes are shocked at the attachment they feel to their babies. This devotion is a right-brain instinctive or intuitive feeling, rather than a left-brain learned, rational response (see Figure 1.1). These women are devastated by the thought of leaving the baby with somebody else while they go back to work. On the other hand, some women have no choice but to return to work, sometimes as early as four to six weeks after the baby is born. If they do not, they may lose their job, and many households cannot exist on one income alone. Only on rare occasions can the father stay home full time for several months to care for a new baby while the mother goes back to work. The guilt in going back to work combined with the enormous expense of full-time day-care is a very powerful stressor.

This career dilemma is a stress-laden problem for parents in the nineties. However, as employers come to realize that family life has a very important effect on the lives of their employees, many companies are coming up with worthwhile and creative approaches in order to alleviate this dilemma. Some companies are experimenting with the creation of half-time or shared jobs for new mothers so that the new mother can keep her job but only work half the time for the first year of her baby's life. Many more companies have day-care centers on the premises so that mothers can nurse their new babies during the work day. Balancing one's job and one's family life is certainly a very important issue.

Super-Mom Syndrome

You want the best of everything in your life, especially for your children. But you are only human, and you will reach the end of your rope at one time or another. Playing the mom role and playing the super-mom role are two entirely different things. Super mom does everything right—she solves all the problems for her family, she works, she raises a family, she has endless energy and enthusiasm—and she is completely out of balance. She is always doing and giving, but she doesn't *take*. Eventually super mom will burn out and become very resentful because she is living a totally unbalanced life. Once you establish that you are going to *give and take* in various proportions, you can truly enjoy your life and your new role to the fullest extent.

SELF-MANAGEMENT FOR STRESS REDUCTION

You have the ability to react to your parenting experiences on many different levels and in a variety of ways. You also have the ability to teach yourself how to react better and how to effectively deal with powerful reactions. The Positive Parenting Fitness program, which is designed to keep you and your new baby healthy and strong, offers some specific techniques to help you control your thoughts and emotions.

You may be overwhelmed by feelings of stress since the arrival of your baby and the changes this has caused in your life. This is a good time to explore a holistic or multifaceted approach for handling the situation. Outline the aspects of your life that need to be analyzed and changed so that you can better cope with stressors. Now consider how and when the following stress management techniques can be applied to reduce stress in your life:

- regular daily exercise

- healthful postpartum nutrition

- letting-go techniques, such as controlled breathing

- self-awareness and faith in yourself

- personal planning and resetting priorities

TALK YOUR WAY TO SELF-AWARENESS

Support Groups

Positive Parenting Fitness classes were initiated ten years ago because a young, frustrated mother, who had been in my pregnancy fitness class, asked me to organize an exercise/support class for postpartum women. The classes combine safe, sensible exercises for you and your baby with a discussion period. Women meet and talk to other new mothers and babies in similar situations. Shared experiences lead to friendships that may go on for years.

If you have a Positive Parenting Fitness class in your community, I would urge you and your baby to sign up immediately. If there is no class in your community, call up your local La Leche leader or ask your pediatrician if there are any parenting support groups available in your area. Just talking to other adults again, after spending all of your time with baby, may be a very worthwhile experience. Although many of your problems will not have definitive answers, talking about how you feel with sympathetic, understanding mothers may be just what you need. Even if you don't think you need a parenting support group, attend one meeting and see what that group is focused on. You may be happily surprised at the practical coping suggestions that arise when a whole group of new mothers meets. Seeking out a support group is not an admission of failure in your new motherhood role. It's a practical action that will help you settle in your role more easily and with more confidence.

Peer Counseling

If you don't have the time or are unable to find a support group, try to find a friend (or even your mate) and do some peer counseling. Peer counseling occurs when one person is the listener and one person is the talker. The listener *only* listens while reassuring the talker through eye contact, gestures, and encouraging words such as, "Tell me more," "Tell me about that," or "Give me the details." The listener may ask questions such as, "How does that make you feel?" The listener can give reassuring hugs or comfort to the talker.

When you are engaged in peer counseling, you should adhere to certain established practices. The following guidelines provide an outline to insure success:

1. When you want someone to listen to you, make sure the person has the time and is willing. You can use the telephone for peer counseling.
2. Set a specific amount of time for the peer-counseling session and stick to it. For example, if you have forty-five minutes, you can divide the time either in half or into twenty-minute segments with a five-minute break for switching roles. A person who gets very emotional may need a few minutes in order to switch roles.
3. You should agree on confidentiality. Whatever happens during a session should be held in confidence.
4. As a listener, you need to recognize that your partner is talking for emotional release. You should not take what you hear too seriously. Don't feel you have to be a psychologist, just be a friend who wants to listen.
5. When you are the listener, remember your role. *Don't interrupt, give advice, or offer an opinion.* Really put your heart and soul into just listening, and become a good listener. With practice, this gets easier and easier.
6. It is important to remain in a positive state of mind when you listen. Don't judge or evaluate your friend's actions. Try to keep your own values out of the counseling.
7. When it is your turn to talk, talk freely, and try to figure out what's really bothering you.
8. Don't be afraid to feel deeply and cry, get angry, feel afraid, or get embarrassed. According to peer-counseling practitioners, there is nothing bad or wrong about really expressing your feelings. It is highly therapeutic. Crying is a natural release of tension. Your baby does it all the time, why shouldn't you do the same thing?
9. Peer-counseling skills can be very useful to open communication with your partner.

CONTROLLED BREATHING: DO IT RIGHT AND LEARN TO RELAX

You would think, with all the ups and downs of new parenting, that you would have to learn hundreds of techniques to become calm and centered or to become revitalized.

However, your body has a set of controls that you can learn to use easily and effectively to reduce your overall stress levels. What is this secret mechanism you possess? It's your breath! Focusing all of your attention on your body's natural breathing process for only a few minutes a day will produce amazing results while flattening your tummy at the same time.

The Physiology of Breathing

In order to take a really deep breath, you have to learn how to relax and use your abdominal muscles. Breathing with a tight tummy shrinks your body's air capacity, thereby allowing your diaphragm and rib muscles to grow weak while leaving the blood hungry for oxygen. Breathing in this way also puts more stress on the body; you have to take two or three shallow breaths to equal the amount of oxygen taken in with one deep abdominal breath.

Some basic knowledge of your body's physiology will help you to understand the different processes involved when you take an abdominal breath. The parts of your body that are most directly involved in the breathing process are the nose (through which air travels), the trachea or windpipe (the connecting link to the lungs), and the lungs (where oxygen is exchanged for carbon dioxide with each breath). The heart and lungs are located in the thorax (chest cavity). The diaphragm (a thick muscle) forms the floor of the thorax. Below the thorax and the diaphragm is the abdominal area of your body, which contains the organs of digestion, reproduction, and excretion. Figure 2.1 illustrates the abdominal breathing sequence.

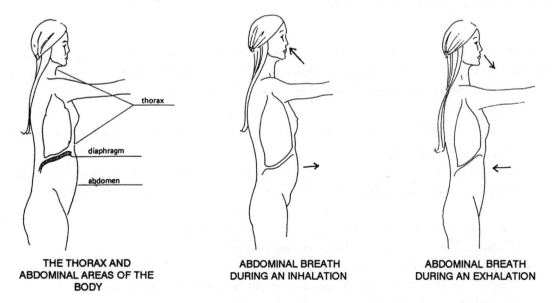

THE THORAX AND ABDOMINAL AREAS OF THE BODY

ABDOMINAL BREATH DURING AN INHALATION

ABDOMINAL BREATH DURING AN EXHALATION

Figure 2.1   Abdominal Breathing Sequence

When you consciously relax the abdominal muscles and inhale, the diaphragm moves downward, thereby increasing your lung capacity. At the same time, there is a reduction of air pressure in the lungs, and fresh air is forced into the lungs because of a vacuum-like pull. With the diaphragmatic downstroke, the interior organs of the abdomen receive a gentle massage, which helps improve digestion and circulation. When exhaling, you have to slightly contract the abdominal wall. This will cause the diaphragm to return to a domed position pushing upward, and will expel carbon dioxide from your lungs.

Breathing and Your Well-Being

Poor breathing habits can have a very negative effect on your body and emotions. Shallow (or upper chest) breathing usually leads to illness and can be accompanied by mental depression. In times of high emotion and sadness you may have noticed that your breathing is very ragged and uneven. When you feel depressed, you may lower your head and let your shoulders sag, thereby lessening your lung capacity. The more you cut down your lung capacity, however, the more depressed you will feel. The brain needs three times more oxygen than the rest of the body. No wonder you often make very little sense when you are highly emotional and upset! At such times, it is important to remember that the full responsibility for your emotional state is in your hands, or "lungs."

Guidelines for Practicing Breathing

The idea of "practicing breathing" may seem very strange to you, since you have been doing it all your life without any guidelines. However, in order to derive the most benefit from the following exercises, certain rules should be followed.

- Check with your caregiver—either doctor or midwife—before beginning any breathing exercise program.
- Use your nose for inhaling and exhaling, unless otherwise instructed. The nasal passages will clean, warm, and moisten the air before it enters your lungs and blood system.
- Hold your breath for the time specified. Never overdo.
- Continually focus on your body as you practice.
- Practice each breath at least five to ten times to achieve the desired results. It is the repetition and coordinated mental concentration that will cause you to either revitalize or calm down.

CALMING BREATHS

In order to calm down quickly, you must close your eyes and tune into your body. The following breaths will calm you down while toning your tummy at the same time.

Abdominal Breath

Benefits

- Calms the nerves while revitalizing the body
- Strengthens the abdominal muscles
- Enriches and purifies blood
- Increases resistance to colds and other respiratory conditions

Directions

1. Sitting in a comfortable cross-legged position on your mat, in a chair, or even from your bed, place your right hand on your lower abdomen. Check to see that your head is up straight, your facial muscles are relaxed, and your back is as straight as is comfortable. Figure 2.1 shows the body parts that are involved.
2. Now exhale as completely as you can through your nose.
3. Relax your abdominal muscles and begin to inhale through your nose, sending the air directly to your lower abdominal area. Imagine that you have a bucket in this area that you are filling up with air.
4. As you inhale, move your abdominal area slightly forward and fill your imaginary bucket as full as possible. Keep your shoulders completely still.
5. Once you have completely filled the bucket, which takes from 5-10 seconds, begin to smoothly exhale.

6. As you exhale and empty the bucket, which should take from 5-10 seconds, contract your abdominal muscles, and try to pull them back close to your spine. Squeeze and hold for 5-10 seconds and then release.
7. At first, repeat 5 times and relax. Work up to 10 breaths and stomach contractions.

Cautions and Comments

- Do not practice this breath too fast or you may feel dizzy.
- As you continue to practice filling and emptying your imaginary bucket, you will be able to inhale and exhale for longer periods of time.
- Abdominal Breaths can also be practiced while lying in bed during early postpartum healing exercises (Chapter Nine).
- Once you have gotten used to abdominal breathing, you won't have to keep your right hand on your abdomen.
- Practice this exercise while feeding your baby, while sitting in your car at red lights, during TV commercials, or any time you have a spare moment.
- To hasten the tightening of your abdominal area, hold for a count of 5 after you exhale.
- You must do 5-10 breaths for this exercise to be effective.

2:8:4 Breath (Breathing with Retention)

Benefits

- Very quickly calms jangled nerves
- Increases lung capacity
- Strengthens the breathing mechanism

Directions

1. Arrange yourself in any comfortable position. Exhale completely out of both nostrils. Close your eyes.
2. Inhale for 2 seconds by mentally counting 1-2.
3. Retain the breath for 8 seconds by mentally counting from 1 through 8.
4. Exhale completely as you contract the tummy area for 4 seconds by mentally counting from 1 through 4.
5. Repeat for 10 rounds.

Cautions and Comments

- Breathe evenly when you inhale and exhale.
- Squeeze every bit of oxygen out when you exhale.
- Use both nostrils throughout this exercise.
- This is an excellent exercise to practice during breastfeeding.

Alternate-Nostril Breath

Benefits

- Calms both the body and mind
- Is the key to emotional control
- Gives a feeling of inner serenity
- Can help relieve headaches

Directions for Variation I

1. Sitting in a comfortable position with your back straight, bring your right palm up in front of your face.
2. Bend the fourth and fifth fingers of your right hand. Lightly block your left nostril with these fingers. Leave your right nostril open (see Figure 2.2).
3. Inhale as fully as you can into your right nostril (without straining); close it off with your thumb.

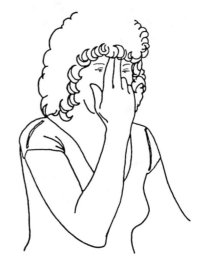

Figure 2.2   Alternate-Nostril Breath

4. Open your left nostril by moving your fourth finger and exhaling completely. The exhalation will usually be longer than the inhalation.

5. Once the exhalation is complete, close off the left side again and begin to inhale with the right.
6. Repeat the procedure for 5 breaths. (Breathe in right and out left, 5 times).
7. After the fifth breath, change the sequence by inhaling with the left and exhaling with the right for 5 breaths.
8. After completing 10 rounds of breaths, rest your hands in your lap, keep your eyes closed, and relax for a while.

Directions for Variation II (with Retention)

1. Begin by following directions 1 and 2 of Variation I.
2. Relax your facial muscles, close your eyes, and begin inhaling smoothly, sending the air to your lower abdomen. When you have inhaled and mentally counted 4 beats, close off the right nostril with your thumb.
3. Hold your breath for a count of 8.
4. Raise your fourth finger and exhale for 4 counts on the left side. Contract your abdomen as you exhale. When the exhalation is complete, close the left side with your fourth finger.
5. Open the right nostril by moving your thumb, and begin to inhale again on the right side for 4 counts. Hold for 8 counts and exhale on the left for 4 counts.
6. Repeat this procedure for 5 rounds on the right side. Then reverse and repeat on the left side for 5 rounds.

Cautions and Comments

- Your hand placement might seem strange for a while, but you will get used to it once you experience the calming effect of the breathing.
- If you have a stuffed nose, you might try inhaling completely through your mouth and then exhaling completely through your nose. These movements will help to temporarily clear out stuffed noses.
- Follow the breath mentally with each inhalation and exhalation.
- You may want to have a tissue handy when practicing this breath.
- Alternate Nostril Breath without retention is an instant headache remedy.
- Have you noticed that you feel calmer already?

Constructive Relaxation Breathing (Your Mini Vacation)

Benefits

- Deeply relaxes the muscles and nervous system
- Releases stored tension and anxieties, thereby restoring a peaceful feeling to your mind and body
- Is a useful energizer
- Helps keep blood pressure within a normal range
- Helps bring joints back into prepregnancy alignment

Directions

1. Lie on your back with your legs placed over a table or chair, as seen in Figure 2.3. Knees should be positioned directly above your hip joint.

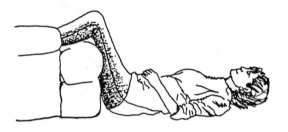

Figure 2.3   Constructive Relaxation
                   Position

2. Rest your hands across your chest or down at your sides. Your head should be aligned with your body.

3. Once you are comfortable, begin to take 10 Abdominal Breaths (page 17).
4. Visualize the two ends of your spine (the top of your neck and your tailbone) moving away from each other.
5. Visualize the front of your pelvis narrowing as the two sides of your pubic bone move closer together.
6. Continue to breathe and relax in this position for 10-20 minutes every day.

Cautions and Comments

• This position is called Constructive Relaxation because it allows you to take a break and let gravity help realign your spine and pelvis while relieving any muscle stress at the same time.
• See Basic Eight (page 136) for more specific relaxation directions and information.

REJUVENATING BREATHS

To rejuvenate your body quickly, you must take in oxygen and then forcefully exhale it using the abdominal muscles. All of these breaths will be highly beneficial for tightening and toning the abdominal area as well as energizing you.

Cleansing Breath

Benefits

• Refreshes and wakes up the mind
• Cleans the lung tissue, which keeps that area of the body healthy
• Helps decongest nasal passages and sinuses
• Strengthens the abdominal area, the lungs, and the diaphragm.

Directions

1. Sit up straight in a chair or get into a cross-legged position. Exhale completely through both nostrils.
2. Inhale using your nose, taking in only one third of a lungful of air while expanding your tummy area forward.
3. With a very strong movement, sud-

denly and quickly pull in the tummy area while exhaling through your nose.

4. Relax and let the air quickly fill up one third of your lungs again.
5. Repeat 10 breaths. Each breath should take about 2 seconds to practice.
6. End with Abdominal Breath (page 17).

Cautions and Comments

• This is an invaluable breath when you have trouble getting out of bed in the morning because you have been up half the night.

• You can increase the rounds of Cleansing Breaths, but always practice 10 rounds followed by an Abdominal Breath (page 17), and then start another round of 10.
• You may want to have a tissue handy when practicing this breath.
• If you feel dizzy or light-headed, reduce the number of breaths you are doing.
• Practice in the car, while doing the dishes, or in any place you wouldn't mind being discovered becoming a choo-choo train.

Charging Breath

Benefits

• Immediate revitalization of body and mind
• Cleans lungs of unwanted residue
• Increases the supply of oxygen to the bloodstream
• Strengthens the lungs, diaphragm, and abdomen

Directions

1. Sit in a chair or in a comfortable cross-legged position with your back and head up straight.
2. Exhale completely. Inhale forcefully, pushing your abdomen out as you inhale.
3. Exhale forcefully (through the nose) as you contract the abdominal area.

4. Repeat steps 2 and 3 for 10 rounds.
5. End with Abdominal Breath (page 17).

Cautions and Comments

• At first it will be difficult to coordinate your tummy movements with your inhalations and exhalations, but this should improve with practice.
• Try to increase your speed as you practice, so that you sound like a choo-choo train.
• Try to keep your breathing rhythmic.
• You may want to have a tissue handy when practicing this breath.
• This breath can make you feel very high or tipsy. Don't overdo.
• Practice only once a day until your body is used to this vigorous workout. Gradually add more rounds.

Energizing Single-Nostril Breath

Benefits

- Energizes your body and mind
- Increases alertness while eliminating fatigue
- Strengthens your breathing mechanism
- Improves your concentration skills

Directions

1. Arrange yourself in any comfortable position.
2. Close your left nostril with your right pointer finger.
3. Close your eyes. Inhale and exhale with right nostril, using only the Abdominal Breath (page 17). Do 10 smooth, slow inhalations and 10 even, complete exhalations.
4. As you inhale, think, "Inhale energy one." As you exhale, think, "Exhale tiredness one." Then continue, "Inhale energy two," "Exhale tiredness two," etc., until you reach "ten." It is very important to keep your mental concentration on these thoughts.
5. Relax your right hand and keep your eyes closed as your breathing returns to normal after 10 rounds.
6. Within 5-10 minutes, you will begin to feel revitalized and renewed.

Cautions and Comments

- Do not substitute this breath for sleep when your body is truly tired.
- If you are left-handed, these directions should be reversed. For left-handed people, the dominant nostril is the left one.

MASSAGE YOUR CARES AWAY

Self Massage

If you could see yourself from your body's point of view, you would probably be surprised at the many animated movements, gestures, and faces you make! You take time to talk to and stimulate your baby, why not take some time for yourself—give yourself a stress-reduction acupressure facial massage.

Acupressure Facial, Neck, and Shoulder Massage

Benefits

- Stimulates the natural flow of energy within the face, neck, and shoulders

- Releases tension, fatigue, and worry lines from the facial area
- Stimulates an extra flow of blood to the face, neck, and shoulders to improve your skin

Directions

1. Sitting in a comfortable position, close your eyes and take 1-5 Abdominal Breaths (page 17).
2. Briskly rub your hands and wrists together to activate the flow of energy into your hands.
3. Refer to Figures 2.4 and 2.5 for location of the pressure points stated in the directions that follow.

CHEEKS

4. Begin your massage by rubbing your cheeks with your fingertips. Massage the center of your cheekbones (Pressure Point #1) with your thumbs to clear and revitalize your sinuses. Rub 15-30 seconds. This massage may drain your sinuses.

EYES

5. Massage around your eyes and eye sockets (Pressure Point #2) with your thumbs for 15-30 seconds.
6. Pinch the bridge of your nose with your finger and thumb as you activate Pressure Point #3. Pinch 5-10 seconds to eliminate eye fatigue and to induce clear vision.
7. Press your eyes with the heel of your hand. Palm and rotate your eyes 10 times in each direction.

NOSE

8. Rub the sides of your nose vigorously and then pinch the end. Press Pressure Point #4 to open the nasal cavities and bronchi.
9. Massage around your mouth, gums, and jaw, pressing deeply under your jawbone with your thumbs. This will increase saliva production and prevent double chin.

EARS

10. Massage around ears and temples (Pressure Point #5) for 15-30 seconds. Massage and pull your ears in all directions, which will activate the flow of energy to your entire body.
11. Massage Pressure Point #6 with your thumbs. Then bat your ears with loose fingers.

HEAD

12. Massage your hairline using all your fingers. Then grab and tug handfuls of hair until your scalp tingles. Using loose wrists, pound gently and lightly on your head (about 50 times) in a counterclockwise direction working out from the center.

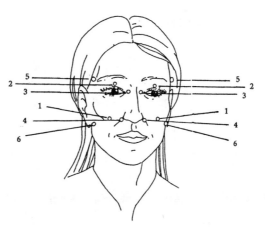

Figure 2.4 Pressure Points of the Face

NECK

13. Massage Pressure Point #6 located under the ridge in the back of the skull. Press in with your thumb and massage for 15–60 seconds.
14. Massage the base of your neck with your thumbs beginning with Pressure Point #7. Massage down the neck to the back, sides, and front.
15. Do two Neck Smiles (page 166), one in each direction.

SHOULDERS

16. Tilt your head to the left and pound your right shoulder with your left fist (keep fist loose). Pound three times from the left neck area to the edge of the shoulder. Repeat on the other side with the opposite hand.
17. Massage Pressure Point #8 by using your left thumb on your right shoulder. Reverse the hand and repeat on the other side.
18. Repeat the same procedure starting from Pressure Point #9. Finish your shoulder massage by inhaling while pressing your shoulders up to your ears, then exhaling while releasing your shoulders.

Cautions and Comments

- You will know you have found the right spot for each pressure point because these areas are highly sensitive. You may feel pain when you first begin to work with each point, but as you massage, these negative sensations should become more pleasurable.

- Using a loose fist to gently pound your body and activate your energy flow is a form of *Do-In* or ancient Chinese acupressure self-massage.

- Rub the different areas of your body until they are warm.

- Try to keep your posture, breathing, and movements as natural yet rigorous as possible.

- You should not feel pain as you work. Ease up if you find certain movements uncomfortable.

- This massage will wake you up and activate your whole body system.

- You can use the same pressure points for a slow, sensual massage.

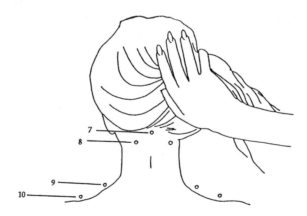

Figure 2.5 Pressure Points of the Neck and Shoulders

A Professional Massage

If you are lucky enough to get a professional massage as a baby gift, you are in for a treat. If not, and if you have the time and the money, this investment in yourself and your well-being can help reduce your stress level, loosen tight muscles, and relax you completely. Most massage therapists work on only one part of the body at a time, while the rest is covered with a sheet. Most play very relaxing music and use scented oils to enhance the feeling of relaxation. Write to the American Massage Therapy Association (AMTA), 1130 West Northshore Ave., Chicago, IL 60626-4670, or call them at (312)472-6782 to find a local AMTA certified therapist.

Some registered massage therapists work with shiatsu or acupressure in addition to massage therapy. Some will even have a portable table and come to your house if you so desire. If you want your spouse to massage you, refer to the section beginning on page 108 for specific directions.

FINDING TIME FOR YOURSELF

Twenty Minutes Does It

When you were pregnant, finding twenty minutes a day for yourself was easy. You simply took the time. Now, with a new baby, finding twenty uninterrupted minutes is almost impossible. I firmly believe that every mother deserves at least twenty minutes a day to do what she wants. You can use this time for a perfume-scented bath, for meditation, for reading a racy novel, or just for sleeping. Your twenty minutes a day should be devoted to accomplishing nothing. Maybe you will choose to have twenty minutes filled with luscious, relaxing music.

Relaxing Music

Calming, relaxing music can put you into a new frame of mind. If you practice Constructive Relaxation Breathing (Your Mini Vacation) found on page 19, you might put on some soothing music while you relax. Focus on the music, letting it deepen your sense of relaxation and of letting go. Over twenty-five musical tapes are suggested on page 310. These audio tapes relax mother as well as baby!

Quick Meditation

With the ups and downs of taking care of your new baby, you may not find consistent time to practice meditation. I learned how to meditate when my sons were quite small. Often they would burst into my washroom (my private meditation room, of course), and climb right on me as I was sitting cross-legged. Even with these kinds of interruptions (and crying babies is in this category), you can do a quick meditation to keep yourself centered and alert.

Heart Centering

Benefits

- Quickly calms you down
- Stops your brain from rampaging
- Quickly recharges and revitalizes you

Directions

1. When you notice that your mind is racing or that you are agitated, **stop.**
2. For a moment, look at yourself as if you were observing another person.
3. Close your eyes and focus your attention on your heart, at the upper center of your body, pumping energy and life throughout your body and brain.
4. Begin to imagine that you can inhale and exhale directly into and out of your heart.
5. Inhale directly into your heart, feeling yourself slow down and center; exhale out of your heart, feeling the bad thoughts and anxieties leaving.
6. Practice 15-20 of these "heartbreaths."
7. Open your eyes and see the world from a new perspective.

Cautions and Comments

- You really need to concentrate on feeling the air going into your heart and then going out again. This concentration will help foster a sense of calm and quiet.
- Your heart is the symbol for your feelings of love, including self-love. This meditation will help these positive feelings grow.

Getting Away From It All

When all else fails, get somebody to watch the baby or take the baby with you and go for a walk outside. If it's cold, bundle up and take the walk anyway. Just the change of scenery, looking at the trees and the flowers, and breathing in fresh air will help you feel better.

Having a "Night on the Town"

At one time or another, you will eventually leave your baby with a babysitter. Trusting another person to take care of your baby is very hard to do, but it is very good for both you and your baby. I can vividly recall leaving my older son, Mat, with my sister for the first time. My husband and I only went to see a movie, but I called from the movie theater to see how Mat was doing. I trusted my sister implicitly, but I had to call anyway.

Going out to dinner, to a movie, or to a show may actually reduce your stress level. When you do something enjoyable away from your baby, you generally return with a fresh outlook. So every now and then, give up the motherhood role for a night and enjoy yourself as a person, not as a mother. You will be better off for it.

A POSITIVE OUTLOOK

There are some simple choices you must make in life. You can either feel sorry for yourself and your situation, or you can take the time and effort to learn how to make your life better. Turning negative things around and looking for the positive sides to them is up to you. Sometimes it's a struggle to find the positive aspects of many adventures in your life, but if you take the time and effort to reshape your body as well as your mind through the techniques described here, you will see life in a more positive way.

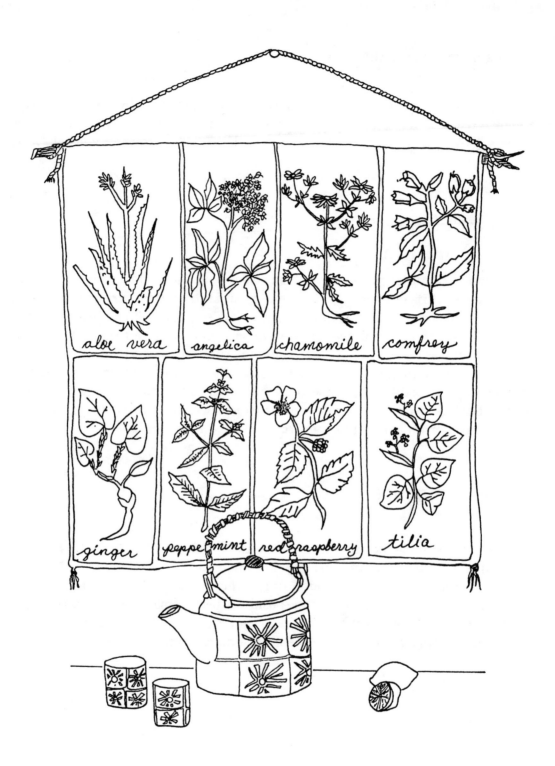

CHAPTER THREE
Remedies for Common Ailments of New Mothers

Have you ever noticed that characters in movies or in television soap operas seldom experience postpartum complaints? These women are thin, shapely, and back to business as usual within a week or two after delivery of their babies. Only rarely do you hear a television character talking about postpartum depression, backache, aching stitches, or engorged breasts. Television's portrayal of life after birth is very unrealistic and is often the cause of unattainable expectations. The reality of the female body for the first six months after the baby's birth needs to be explored and understood.

This chapter discusses some of the most common complaints of postpartum women and some natural remedies for them. These remedies include Positive Parenting Fitness exercises, dietary changes, cleansing and relaxation breathing techniques as well as general information for easing worried minds. Concerns pertaining to sexual readjustment and to the postpartum "blues" are so important that entire chapters are devoted to them.

In this chapter, I hope to answer your questions about and provide explanations for many of your concerns after the baby is born. New parents may have little time or inclination to call a doctor or midwife. Please note that certain postpartum symptoms are serious and need immediate attention. Remember that you are still under the care of your doctor or midwife even though your child has been delivered.

Some information in this chapter is included for peace of mind, especially for first-time mothers. I can still vividly remember looking down at my tummy after the birth of my first son. What I saw resembled a bowl of very jiggly jello. I was shocked. No one had warned me that my body would look like this after having a baby. Then I tried to move this jiggly mass and it didn't move! I remember feeling somewhat depressed and having crying episodes for quite a while. My expectations of a nice, flat, smooth tummy area right after delivery were not fulfilled. It was only after six months of vigorous exercise, long walks, and proper diet that my body returned to its prepregnancy state. I hope my candid writing will prepare you for and help you through this major transitional stage.

Using Herbs

According to Susun S. Weed, herbalist and author of *The Wise Woman Herbal for the Childbearing Year*, herbal tea is made by using one teaspoon of dried herb, such as red raspberry or camomile, per cup of boiling water. Add an extra teaspoon for the pot. Let it steep in your cup or pot for twenty minutes. Enjoy herbal tea plain or with lemon and honey. (Do not give honey to infants.)

Infusions from herbal leaves, such as comfrey, are made by using one ounce of dried leaves (two handfuls of cut-up leaves or three handfuls of whole leaves) in a quart canning jar. Fill the jar to the top with boiling water, put the cover on, and let steep for four hours at room temperature.

More detailed directions are found in Susun Weed's book, which is listed in the Recommended Reading section at the back of this book.

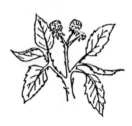

Red Raspberry Leaf
(Rubus Ideaus)

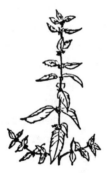

Peppermint
(Mentha Peperita)

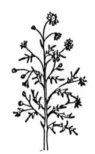

Camomile
(Matricaria or Anthemis Nobilis)

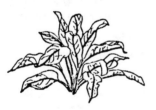

Comfrey
(Symphytum Officinale)

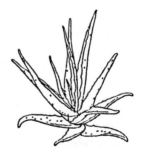

Aloe Vera

Aching Perineal Stitches

Useful Exercises

- Abdominal Breath (page 17)
- Kegels (page 104). Start doing these as soon as the area is stitched.
- The Squeeze (page 122)

Cleansing Techniques

- After going to the bathroom, wash the area with warm water using a squirt or irri bottle. Jeannine Parvati Baker, herbal expert, recommends fresh comfrey or ginger tea in the irri bottle. Carefully pat the healing area dry with a clean wipe or use a blow dryer on the cool setting. Always wipe from front to back so as not to contaminate the wound.
- Soap used too frequently may cause dryness or irritation to the skin and may contribute to bladder infections. Use soap only when bathing or showering.

Cautions

- Try not to use pillows to sit on (although they may be useful the first few days). This is so you will constantly be reminded to do your Kegels.

Tips

- Soak in a warm or cool sitz bath (use 1-2 inches of water) once a day for a few minutes. A sitz bath is taken in a sitting position so bacteria won't be introduced into your vagina. Putting some herbs into your sitz bath, such as ginger for itching or comfrey for healing, is a good idea. Most pharmacies have portable sitz baths that fit inside the toilet and are relatively inexpensive (five to ten dollars).
- While soaking in a sitz bath, close your eyes and visualize a healed perineum.
- Combine 1/2 cup witch hazel and 1/2 cup water. Soak a soft cloth in the mixture and place on the healing area. This is soothing and helps promote healing.
- Boil a handful of dried (or one fresh) comfrey leaves in one cup of water for five minutes. Let the liquid cool. Soak a soft cloth in the liquid; wring out and apply warm or cold. This will soothe the tender tissue. Repeat five times a day.

Cesarean Section Complaints

There are certain complaints common to those women who have had a Cesarean delivery. These complaints are discussed now. Helpful information is also provided to help alleviate these common discomforts.

Incisions

Cleansing

- Wash your hands before and after handling the dressing on your incision to help prevent infection.
- For minimal discomfort, remove the tape on the dressing by pulling in the direction of the incision.
- Wash the incision line with plain water. Do not use soap. Soap can be drying and irritating.
- Pat the incision dry. Apply a clean dressing, making sure not to touch the side of the dressing that will be applied to your incision. Hold dressing in place with one piece of tape.

Cautions

- If your incision gets red or puffy, feels wet, or becomes increasingly more tender, contact your caregiver immediately.
- Call your caregiver if you smell a foul odor of if you see blood, pus, or large amounts of fluid coming from the incision.
- *Do not* use goldenseal on incisions as it may be drying or irritating.
- After the Cesarean (C-section), you may experience discomfort such as pain and a burning sensation at the incision sight. Your caregivers may offer you pain-killing medications in the hospital and for use at home. Use these medications carefully. If you are breastfeeding, your baby will be affected by everything you ingest. Sleep, poor-sucking, slow-feeding infants result when mom takes pain killers.

Tips

- You may experience itching in varying degrees of intensity for several months as your wound heals; this is normal. Relieve it with an olive-based ointment made with calendula, comfrey, or plantain. Such ointments are available at health food stores.
- As your wound heals, it will go through changes in appearance. At first it will be large and reddish-purple in color. There may be areas of bruised skin surrounding the incision. As the color begins to fade, the scar may become raised and bumpy in places. Usually within a few months, the scar will smooth out and become a thin white line. If you have had a "bikini" incision, which falls below your pubic hairline, the scar will be unnoticeable. Calendula ointment insures scar-free healing.
- Minor pain feels worse when you don't get enough rest. Nap whenever you can.

Gas Pains

Useful Exercises

- Head-to-Knee Posture (page 124)
- Abdominal Breath (page 17)
- Pelvic Rocking (page 129)
- Lying on your left side, pull your knees up into your chest, and gently massage your tummy with a circular motion in a counterclockwise manner.
- Rock in a rocking chair while nursing your baby.
- Walk around to move the gas down and out.

Comments

- Discomfort due to gas build-up is quite common after a Cesarean section. Your bowels function more slowly as a result of the anesthesia and your intestines are "grumpy" at having been handled during your surgery.
- Gas pains peak on the second or third day postpartum and are a very positive sign indicating that your intestines are working again.

Tips

- To decrease gas pains, avoid carbonated beverages and drinking through a straw, which increases air intake.

- Avoid foods that cause gas, such as beans and cabbage.
- Drink hot liquids, especially peppermint tea.
- Put 1/4-1/2 teaspoon of powdered ginger in a cup of hot water. Add honey. This "relief" drink usually takes as little as five minutes to work.
- Eat a cup of yogurt or take two to four acidophilus capsules. Relief should occur within five minutes.

Shoulder and Upper-Back Pain

Comments

- Postpartum pain in one or both shoulders and the upper-back area is caused by the collection of air and blood under the diaphram. It is referred through your nervous system to your shoulders and goes away in several days as the blood and air are reabsorbed.
- This pain is the direct result of Cesarean section.
- The pain can also be caused by the strains of pushing during labor and birth.

Tips

- Pain medication might be recommended, but try a hot shower, a cup of hops tea, and/or the application of five drops of skullcap tincture before resorting to drugs.
- A shoulder and back massage can be very helpful.
- Heat applied to aches can also help.

After Pains (Uterine Contractions)

Useful Exercises

- Abdominal Breath (page 17) while the contractions are happening.
- Try to relax the voluntary body muscles while the uterus contracts.
- Walking can help.

Comments

- These are menstrual-type cramps that often occur while you are nursing. They are a good indication that your uterus is shrinking normally.
- These uterine contractions are much more noticeable after the birth of your second or third child and can be more intense than labor pains.
- You will only notice these contractions for two or three days postpartum.

Tips

- Your favorite menstrual-cramp remedy may help.
- Try ginger or catnip tea to relieve after pains.
- A hot water bottle or heating pad over your abdomen may help.

Backaches

Useful Exercises

- The Bridge (page 132)
- Cobra in the Sun Salute (page 157)
- Pelvic Rocking (page 129)
- Sun Salute (page 154)
- See Chapter Fourteen, "Exercises Designed to Relieve Backaches," for back-relief exercises you can do with your baby.

Comments

- Your lower back can be weak from a few weeks to a few months after giving birth due to your stretched abdominal muscles. When your abdominal tone returns, usually twenty-one to twenty-eight days after birth, your back should rapidly improve.
- Adjusting your posture to your new non-pregnant state could take up to six weeks.

Tips

- Slow down your activities. Go at your own pace the first few weeks postpartum. All the work you feel you have to do right now will wait for you!

Bodily Elimination

Useful Exercises

- Deep Abdominal Breaths (page 17)
- The Squeeze (page 122)
- Kegels (page 104)
- Try to take a short walk each day. This form of exercise will help get your system back to normal.

Cleansing

- Cleanse the vaginal area carefully and completely after each elimination.
- Wash with a soft cloth or disposable wipes.
- Apply witch hazel or oil to any hemorrhoids and to your stitched area.

Cautions

- Bran may cause a blockage, especially after a Cesarean section, so its use is *not* recommended.
- If you have a burning sensation when you urinate or have a frequent urge to urinate but pass very little water, drink unsweetened cranberry juice and call your doctor or midwife immediately. You may have cystitis or a urinary tract infection.
- Dark, concentrated urine with a strong odor; or pain in your back, side, or lower abdomen could be the sign of a bladder infection. Call your caregiver immediately.

Tips

- Be sure to eat fresh vegetables, stewed fruit, and whole grains. This diet will help eliminate constipation.
- Drink two to three quarts of liquid a day in the form of water, milk, fruit juices, and herbal teas.
- According to Susun Weed, herbalist, Vitamin C is helpful for acidifying the urine and washing out harmful bacteria. Doses up to 500 mgs per hour can be used effectively. Large doses of Vitamin C can cause loose bowel movements.

- Soak in a portable sitz bath or your bathtub to soothe the urethra area.
- Pour some warm water on the urethra to induce urination.
- For comfort, you can urinate in the sitz bath. Then cleanse the perineum thoroughly.
- Try standing in the shower when you urinate. This way you won't irritate your stitches.

Breast Infection (Mastitis)

Comments

- If your breasts are tender with a reddened area; if your entire breast is hot, hard, and swollen; if you have a fever, chills, nausea, or aching pain similar to the flu, you probably have mastitis.

Cautions

- If you have the symptoms of mastitis, notify your caregiver immediately.
- Breast infections are almost always caused by too little rest. *Sleep when your baby sleeps* or take fifteen-minute naps every two hours.

Tips

- Submerge your entire breast in a small bowl filled with hot water for two or three minutes.
- Apply hot parsley compresses (see Engorged or Painful Breasts, page 39) at least four times a day. Jeannine Parvati Baker, herbalist, recommends violet leaf compresses.
- Nurse on the infected breast for as long as possible at least every three hours during the day and when the baby wakes at night.
- Your breast infection won't make your baby ill. Baby may not like the taste of the milk from the infected breast so offer this breast first in feeding when baby is hungriest and less likely to be picky.

Clogged Milk Ducts

Comments

- Symptoms of clogged milk ducts include small, red, tender lumps on the breasts; red streaks radiating out from the lumps; breast swelling; and acute pain.

Cautions

- Continue nursing on the breast that has a plugged or blocked duct. Discontinuing to nurse will increase your discomfort and endanger your milk supply.

Tips

- As soon as you notice symptoms, nurse more frequently and for longer periods of time. Change your baby's position often during feedings.
- Hand express or use a breast pump if your baby doesn't empty milk from breasts.
- Right before nursing, apply a warm herbal compress. Place a handful of freshly chopped, or dried and crumbled herb leaves in a clean cotton diaper or cloth. Try comfrey, parsley, yarrow, plantain, daisy, or violet leaves. Tie the cloth with a rubber band and steep in simmering water for ten to fifteen minutes. Cool until the temperature feels comfortable, then compress the affected breast with this hot, wet bundle.
- Try an herbal soak. Allow the preceding herbal solution to cool even more, then pour the mixture into a small bowl, leaving enough room to submerge the breast in. Let soak in the liquid for as long as is comfortable. Repeat several times a day.
- Try to get plenty of rest. A good sleep will usually clear the clogged duct within a few hours or overnight at the most.
- Be in touch with your caregiver.

Engorged or Painful Breasts

Comments

- If you don't nurse, engorgement will usually occur between the third and seventh day postpartum. Your breasts will feel hard and tender and may look like large balls. Take heart, this will only last one or two days.

Cautions

- Nurse your baby often during the first few days after birth to get the colostrum flowing. This will prevent engorgement.
- Nurse your baby at least every two to three hours of the day during your first six weeks postpartum.

Tips

- Wear a nursing bra twenty-four hours a day. Make sure it is not too tight for you.
- A self-breast massage in a hot shower can be helpful. Place one hand under the breast and the other hand on the top of the breast; slowly and smoothly massage toward the nipple. Use the same massaging movement on the sides of the breast. Repeat on the other breast until the breasts relax and the milk begins to flow.
- Be sure to drink two to three quarts of liquid a day: water, milk, fruit juice, and herbal teas. It's easy to do if you drink a cup before and another during or after nursing.
- Ice packs or heat can often help. Try hot herbal compresses (see page 38). Use the method that feels best to you.
- A warm shower where you apply a very hot towel or washcloth to the breasts will get the milk to flow and relieve engorgement. You can also submerge your breast in a bowl of hot water for three to five minutes.
- To get the milk flowing, you can use an electric, battery-operated, or manual breast pump. Hand expressing is also effective.

Sore or Cracked Nipples

Comments

- If your nipples are persistently or suddenly sore, you might suspect a thrush infection. Symptoms of thrush are pink, flaky skin and itchy nipples. Coat the nipples with yogurt or use plantain compresses.

Cautions

- Avoid using alcohol, soap, and perfumed creams on your breasts or nipples
- Make sure you correctly place your baby to your breast. Hold your baby in the crook of your arm with your hand on your baby's buttocks or upper thigh. Make sure that the baby's buttocks is at the same height as the breast. Use pillows on your lap for support. Hold your breast by placing four fingers beneath it and your thumb on top, making a letter "C." Make sure that your hand is *not* on the areola (dark area). *Do not use the cigarette-hold position.* Tilting the nipple up will incorrectly position your nipple in the baby's mouth, thus causing sore nipples. Make sure that at least one-half inch of the areola is in the baby's mouth and that the nipple is centered. Bring the baby to the breast. *Don't bring the breast to the baby!*

Tips

- Gently massage your own milk into your nipples
- You can apply crushed ice in a wet cloth or in a wet, frozen gauze pad immediately before and after nursing. Ice will ease the pain of sore nipples.
- Applying Vitamin-E oil very sparingly after nursing will help to heal and strengthen your nipples.
- Four or five times a day, apply hot comfrey or parsley compresses for five minutes (see Clogged Milk Ducts, page 38).
- Apply the clear gel from a fresh aloe vera leaf to heal and soothe cracked nipples. Be sure to wash it off before nursing your baby because the taste is quite bitter.
- Expose your breasts to the air. Wear your nursing bra with the flaps down whenever possible.
- Use a warm or cool blow dryer on your nipples after feeding.
- Expose your breasts to sunlight or shine a 40-watt bulb on your breasts for five to ten minutes a day.
- If problems persist, contact your caregiver, your local La Leche League leader, or a lactation consultant.

Depression

Useful Exercises

- Abdominal Breath with Retention (page 18)
- Alternate Nostril Breath (page 18)
- Cobra in the Sun Salute (page 157)
- Shoulderstand (page 144)
- Sun Salute (page 154)
- Take a nice, long, leisurely walk; walk with your baby in a carriage or in a front-pack carrier.

Comments

- Some feelings of depression are a natural part of the postpartum period. The big event is over and the real work has begun.
- Postpartum depression is related to the rapid hormonal readjustment in your body after your baby is born.
- An in-depth discussion of postpartum depression appears in Chapter Four.

Cautions

- If your depression is long-lasting and severe, call your doctor or midwife.
- Too much company during the first three weeks postpartum can cause some feelings of depression. You may be too tired to entertain your company or you may find the company stays too long.

Tips

- Check your diet to see that it includes enough foods containing B vitamins. This would include foods such as sunflower or pumpkin seeds, brewer's yeast, eggs, beef liver, blackstrap molasses, and whole grain cereals.
- One or two cups of lemon balm tea with milk and honey may relieve mild depression.
- Jeannine Parvati Baker, herbalist, recommends borage tea.
- Ask yourself who or what are you angry at or about.
- According to Susun S. Weed in *Wise Woman Herbal for the Childbearing Year,* "Breastfeeding is probably the best cure for postpartum depression. The process

helps moderate hormonal swings, increases the endorphin level, and allows your body to regain hormonal balance slowly and evenly."
- Discuss your feelings with your mate.
- Try to find other women in your area with whom you can discuss your feelings.
- For about the first six weeks, nap when the baby naps, and keep your phone off the hook.
- Try to give and get a regular massage.

Hair Fallout

Useful Exercises

- Fish (page 149)
- Shoulderstand (page 144)

Comments

- Do not be discouraged if you have a bathroom sink full of hair. This is a natural postpartum experience.
- It is natural for hair to become thinner and sparser after pregnancy and childbirth. Normally you lose 50-100 hairs each day. Pregnancy often slows this loss. Many women find that their hair grows better than normal during pregnancy. Once the baby is born, your hormonal levels drop and hair loss begins. You are actually shedding hair that should have been lost during pregnancy.

Cautions

- If hair fallout persists after six months, check with your caregiver.

Fatigue

Useful Exercises

- Alternate Nostril Breathing (page 18)
- Chest Expander (page 251)
- Cleansing Breath (page 20)
- Constructive Relaxation (page 19)
- Sitting Spinal Twist (page 140)

Comments

- Some physical and mental exhaustion during the weeks after birth is natural.
- The major causes of postpartum exhaustion include the physical effort of labor and birth; dramatic changes in your body as it begins to return to its nonpregnant state; hormonal changes when you breastfeed; changing emotions as you take on a new role; taking care of a newborn; and, of course, lack of rest.

Cautions

- If you give birth in a hospital, try to return home as soon as possible. Hospitals are not restful places.
- Do not rely on candy for quick energy. This will pep you up temporarily, but you will feel just as tired when the "sugar high" wears off.
- Try to limit your visitors. If necessary, use the excuse that this is the order of your doctor or midwife.

Tips

- Try to make arrangements to have help when you get home from the hospital.
- Share responsibilities with your mate for the care of your newborn.
- *Sleep when your baby sleeps* (see page 57). If you can, take your phone off the hook when you and your baby are napping. Remember to put the phone back on the hook once you've gotten up again.
- Make arrangements to spend at least twenty minutes a day by yourself.
- Eat often, choosing easily digested and nourishing foods.
- Eat high-protein snacks such as cottage cheese, fish, peanut and sunflower seed mixtures, and cheese and crackers. They are good for sustained energy.

Fever

Cautions

- A spiking fever or a fast-rising fever are warning signs of infection. Call your caregiver immediately.
- A fever of 101° F or higher on any two of the first ten postpartum days (except for the day of the actual birth) can be a sign of Birth Fever. Check with your caregiver; you may have to be treated with a prescription drug.

Tips

- Do not practice any exercises when you have a fever.
- Increase your intake of fluids and of foods that are rich in protein, Vitamin B (whole grains, sunflower and pumpkin seeds, eggs), and Vitamin C (broccoli, citrus fruits, green and red peppers).

Flabby Stomach

Useful Exercises

- Abdominal Breath with Retention (page 18)
- The Bridge (page 132)
- Half Sit-Ups (page 123)
- Single Leg Lifts (page 125)
- Sitting Spinal Twist (page 140)
- Stomach Lift (page 139). *Wait three weeks before beginning this exercise.*
- Taking a one-mile walk each day will help get the tone back into this area.

Comments

- Don't feel depressed when you look at your tummy and see loose, flabby muscles. It took nine months to expand and it is going to take a reasonable period of time (from three to six months) to become truly flat again.
- Muscle tone normally returns to the tummy area anywhere from fourteen to twenty-eight days after the baby is born. Until that time, it is really hard to pull in

the tummy muscles. Keep trying!
- Breastfeeding on demand often helps flatten your stomach.
- If you started your pregnancy with a loose tummy area, now is the time to work on getting it tight again.

Headaches

Useful Exercises

- Acupressure Massage (page 22)
- Alternate Nostril Breath (page 18). Do ten rounds in an upright position.
- Complete Relaxation (page 152) for ten to twenty minutes a day.
- Neck Smiles (page 166)

Cautions

- Cut down on dairy products in your diet. Dairy products can cause excess mucus, sinus problems, and headaches.
- Consult your caregiver if you experience a severe, long-lasting headache.
- Minimize your consumption of caffeine products such as coffee, tea, colas, and cocoa. Caffeine dilates blood vessels and then constricts them, which causes headaches.
- Avoid foods with MSG (monosodium glutamate), which is often found in Chinese food and foods with nitrates, such as luncheon meats. Both MSG and nitrates can cause headaches in sensitive people.
- Avoid alcoholic beverages including wine and champagne.

Tips

- Try a cup of strong peppermint, rosemary, catnip, or sage tea.
- Do not sleep with your head under the covers, for this creates a shortage of oxygen, which can then cause a headache.
- Tight jaw muscles can cause migraine headaches. Are your jaw and neck muscles relaxed? Massage can help relieve strain (see page 22).
- Make Abdominal Breaths part of your daily routine. Consciously controlling your breathing can often prevent and eliminate headaches.
- For sinus headaches, press hot towels on your head and face while you stand un-

a hot shower. Lightly massage sinus areas on forehead and cheeks to stimulate drainage of sinuses.

- Sometimes ice packs placed at the base of your neck, over your sinus areas, and over your eyes can be very helpful in reducing pain. Try alternating hot and cold packs.

Hemorrhoids

Useful Exercises

- The Squeeze (page 122). Coordinate your breathing when practicing the Squeeze. *Exhale*: Lock the anal muscles and hold for as long as you can hold your breath. *Inhale*: Release the muscles. Repeat this coordinated sequence five to ten times as often during the day as you can. Practice the Squeeze in the shower. Fold a washcloth until it is a small rectangle. Wet the cloth then wring it out. Place the washcloth on the hemorrhoidal area and practice the Squeeze. You should be able to hold the washcloth there. Relax the muscles and let the washcloth drop. Repeat from five to ten times.
- Shoulderstand (page 144) and the Squeeze practiced together

Cautions

- Raw vegetables and bran flakes may cause bleeding if your intestinal tissue is swollen or torn.

Tips

- Increase roughage in your diet to soften stools and make elimination easier. Foods that increase roughage are: fresh and dried fruits, cereals, and prune juice.
- Soaking in a sitz bath several times a day does wonders for hemorrhoids. You can buy a sitz bath at most pharmacies or surgical supply stores or use a shallow wash basin. Good herbal infusions to sit in include witch hazel bark, yarrow flowers, oak bark, plantain, or comfrey leaves.
- Some women prefer soaking in a bathtub. Add two quarts herbal infusion to the bath water. Use the time for Complete Relaxation (page 152).
- Apply Vitamin-E cream or oil to the anal area after it has been thoroughly cleaned and dried.

•Use cold compresses of witch hazel three times a day.
•Keep your feet and legs elevated on a stool while eliminating. This will help the bowels move by releasing the anal muscles.

Lochia (Vaginal Flow or Discharge)

Comments

•Lochia is a result of the body's natural cleansing method. It is the discharge of blood, mucus, and tissue (which may appear as clots) from your uterus. This flow cleans out the uterus and enables it to shrink back to its prepregnancy size.
•As approximately four pounds of uterine muscle (the amount made while you were pregnant) must be broken down, the lochia may be copious and may go on for days.
•Lochia is not dirty or foul-smelling; it is similar to menstrual blood.
•Lochia should be viewed as part of the natural healing process.
•At first this discharge will resemble your menstrual flow. Then it will turn brown, then yellow, then white, and finally, colorless.
•Usually your lochia will last from two to six weeks.
•After having a Cesarean section, you will have the same lochia as you would have had after a vaginal delivery.

Cautions

•During this time of bodily cleansing, be sure that you are still taking prenatal vitamins plus iron.
•If the lochia becomes excessive, turns bright red, or has a foul odor call your caregiver immediately.
•If the blood turns from brown to bright red or increases in quantity, it is a sign that you are doing too much and you should rest.
•If you soak two sanitary napkins within thirty minutes, call your doctor or midwife. Sit down or get into bed immediately.

Tips

•Include iron-rich foods in your diet such as liver, prune juice, molasses, peanuts, and apricots. These foods will help you keep your energy level high.

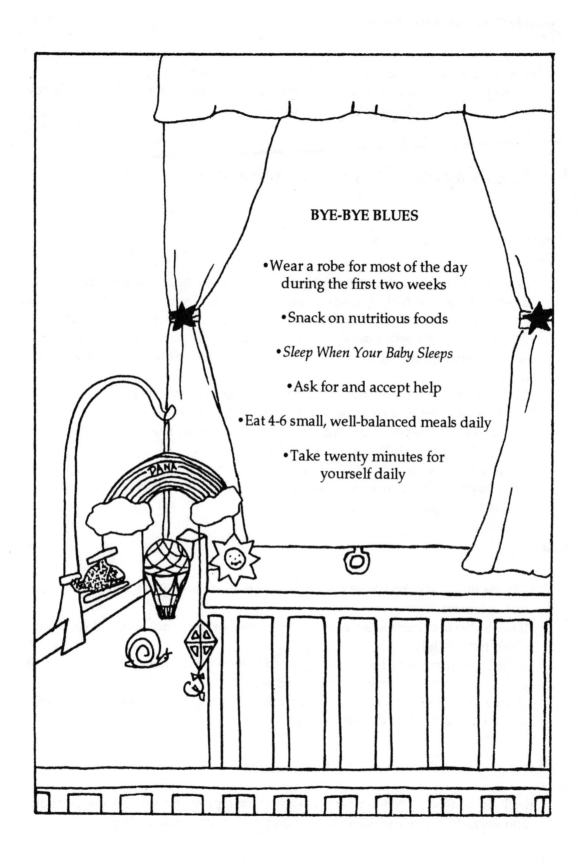

BYE-BYE BLUES

- Wear a robe for most of the day during the first two weeks

- Snack on nutritious foods

- *Sleep When Your Baby Sleeps*

- Ask for and accept help

- Eat 4-6 small, well-balanced meals daily

- Take twenty minutes for yourself daily

CHAPTER FOUR

Understanding and Coping with the "Blues"

Betty was a happy, positive, twenty-six-year-old married woman with a precocious two-year-old son. Three days before the arrival of her second child she was hospitalized with pneumonia. She returned home after two days of oxygen and intravenous feedings. Her husband was called out of town on business the day after her return from the hospital. That same evening, ten days ahead of schedule, she went into labor. Her sister, who was only vaguely familiar with the breathing exercises for labor and birth, was able to help Betty through labor. Betty missed her husband and found relaxing difficult, but after a short, four-hour labor, she gave birth to a healthy baby girl. Betty only bonded a few minutes with her new daughter before the nurses whisked the newborn off to the nursery. When Betty's husband arrived at the hospital the next afternoon, she was overjoyed to see him. She wanted to go home as quickly as possible so that her whole family could be together. As she put it, "I wanted to prove that we could do it alone with out my mother and the family helping."

After arriving home, Betty found that the first few days went well. Then, unexpectedly, there was a severe change. Betty continues, "At that time, my crying started—that was okay at first to deal with—until it got much worse instead of better. One night I was with the kids and was doing the dishes. All of a sudden, I had a tremendous fear of dying. The feeling was so overwhelming, I was really frightened. I felt as if everything I had was going to be taken away from me or that I was going to leave. It was a very sick feeling. Along with these feelings, I had strange thoughts about my children. Christopher [her son] seemed to have grown up very fast, and I kept thinking that he was already in school and no longer needed me. At the same time, I was feeling very detached from him. We were like strangers. I would cry even when he hugged and kissed me. My feelings for the new baby were very negative. I felt she was an intruder. I cried because I realized that Christopher would never nurse again. My thoughts and feelings seemed totally irrational, yet very real at the time."

It was while she was in this frame of mind that Betty and her new baby came to my Positive Parenting Fitness class. Something had obviously changed the perky, positive woman I had come to know in my pregnancy fitness class. Betty looked tired and run down, her face held little expression, there were tears in her eyes, and she was extremely nervous. I asked Betty if she realized that she was probably experiencing postpartum depression. "No," she replied. I then asked her if she knew what had led up to this physical and emotional state. Again, her response was, "No."

There are different theories about what causes the baby blues (see page 56). According to a recent study conducted by British pediatrician Aidan Macfarlane, these blues occur in about 60 percent of mothers who give birth in hospitals, while only in 16 percent of mothers who give birth at home. According to Helen Varney of the Maternal-Newborn Program at Yale University School of Nursing, postpartum blues are largely a psychological phenomenon of the woman who is separated from her baby and her family. It would seem, then, that the birth setting can have a profound impact on a woman's experience of new motherhood. Betty's story clearly supports this theory.

If possible, try to keep your baby with you during the first hours after birth. It may well be that your instinctive right-brain (page 6) takes over during the hours after giving birth; when these instinctive needs are not met, the "blues" occur. There are many other factors that may contribute to the blues. These will be discussed in detail in this chapter.

DIET AND POSTPARTUM BLUES

The importance of a well-balanced diet to your general well-being the first days after your baby is born cannot be emphasized enough. This nutritional emphasis must begin even before your baby is born if you are to have the stamina necessary for labor and birth. In Betty's case, she had lost her appetite with the onset of pneumonia, which resulted in a poorly nourished body. Important B vitamins and iron were lacking; this lack probably contributed to her feelings of depression.

The excitement of childbirth may temporarily put your appetite out of commission, but try to remember, for your sake and your baby's, that you must eat well and often. Encourage your family and friends to bring you fruits, nuts, muffins, and breads rather than sugar-laden chocolates and cakes. Highly recommended snack foods include dried fruits (especially prunes and apricots); sunflower, pumpkin, and sesame seeds; nuts; and cheese and crackers.

As soon as you begin to eat again after giving birth, be sure to eat raw fruits and vegetables, and drink plenty of water in order to avoid constipation. If you give birth in a hospital, you will be encouraged to have a bowel movement before being discharged. Since the perineal area is often sutured and quite tender after the birth of the baby, constipation problems can only make matters more painful and depressing.

Vitamin Deficiency

In times of overwhelming excitement, the body immediately burns any B and C vitamins that are on hand. Since these vitamins cannot be made or stored within the body once the supply is depleted, a person may begin to experience a depressed mental state. It is, therefore, extremely important to include foods rich in B and C vitamins in your diet. B-rich-vitamin foods include brown rice; cracked wheat; sunflower, pumpkin, and sesame seeds; buckwheat groats; oats; millet; wheat germ; and cottage cheese. Liver is a wonderful source of both B and C vitamins. Citrus fruits and dark yellow fruits and vegetables (oranges, papaya, cantaloupe, yellow squash) are also a good source of Vitamin C.

When my husband came to visit me after the birth of our first son, Mat, he brought a brown paper bag. I opened the bag and found six ripe, juicy nectarines. My husband knew what I needed to eat at that time better than I did! And I have the perfect graduation gift for my Positive Pregnancy Fitness students; to assure them plenty of B vitamins after the baby is born, I give out pink and blue bags of raw sunflower seeds.

Iron Deficiency

Another vitally important mineral during postpartum is iron. In a recent medical study based upon 1,000 deliveries, it was found that 20 percent of the new mothers were suffering from anemia or lack of iron by the fourth day postpartum. In 5 percent of these women it was very severe. The major symptom of iron deficiency is weakness or tiredness. Since it is usual to feel both tired and weak after the physical exertion of having a baby, it's important to eat iron-rich foods such as liver, beans, spinach, blackstrap molasses, and split peas. An eight-ounce glass of prune juice contains 10.5 milligrams of iron (10-15 milligrams is necessary to maintain good health). Continue taking your prenatal vitamins and/or iron supplements during the postpartum period. Eating foods rich in Vitamin C, such as red and green peppers and liver, for example, will boost your iron absorption.

Diet and the Nursing Mother

If you are nursing your baby, an additional 500 calories should be added to your diet, as well as one extra serving of calcium per day for milk production. Without this, the baby will be taking what she needs at your expense. The first few days after delivery are not the right time to go on a weight-reduction diet. (Refer to the information found in Chapter Five for safely losing weight.) You may be looking at yourself in the mirror after your shower and become discouraged by what you see. Remember, however, that it took nine full months for your body to grow and expand, and it is going to take a reasonable amount of time (probably at least nine months) for you to regain your prepregnancy shape. The first few weeks postpartum is a time to focus on settling into your new role; it is a time of nights without sleep, new routines, and new demands. If you let yourself get run down at this time, you will most probably experience the "blues."

TIREDNESS AFTER BIRTH

According to a recent study conducted at the University of Iowa, researchers found the most common time for new moms to suffer with bouts of fatigue is approximately two weeks after giving birth. This is largely due to lack of sleep coupled with the new set of infant-care demands. This research may only confirm what you already know!

Please keep the tips found on page 57 in mind during those first critical weeks after giving birth. Make sure to yawn when you want your company to leave, wear your robe, and make sure you *sleep when your baby sleeps.*

VISITORS AND THE "BLUES"

Once your baby is born, family and friends will begin to focus their attention on the baby rather than on you. Throughout your pregnancy, you were the main interest; now, all or most questions and concerns are about the baby. This loss of attention can be a let-down for some women, causing a "blue" period. If you have these feelings, face them, evaluate them, and finally accept them. Use Abdominal Breathing (page 17) to calm and center your mind when these thoughts occur. Alternate Nostril Breathing (page 18) can help prevent any headaches that result from tension or anxiety. Taking walks with your baby is a great stress reducer. It's important to be aware that these uncomfortable feelings are a natural part of the postpartum period; strangely enough, this seems to help.

Once you are settled at home with your baby, your family and friends will want to visit. You will want your guests to see the baby and you will want to be a gracious hostess as well. However, this is not the appropriate time to prove yourself in this area. Remember that *rest is one of the key elements of a good postpartum adjustment.* A quick way to insure a case of the "blues" is by having too much company for long periods of time in the early weeks after the baby is born. Visiting with friends can be very tiring. Tactfully tell your family and friends that visits right after the baby is born need to be short. If you have time during the last weeks of pregnancy, bake some nutritious muffins or breads, then wrap and freeze them. When company comes, tell them where to find these refreshments, where your coffee or tea pots are located, and let them serve you as well as themselves. Using paper plates is also helpful. It is essential to keep your socializing to a minimum during the first two to three weeks postpartum.

TIME MANAGEMENT

It may come as a shock for first-time mothers to realize just how many hours are spent taking care of a new baby. Any routine that you followed prior to the birth will have to be distinctly altered; basic priorities will have to be changed. It is common for many new mothers to get discouraged because they feel they are not doing anything other than taking care of the baby! Often their fantasy of what living with a new baby was going to be like and the reality of the situation are not similar at all. Any time you find yourself thinking, "I haven't done anything around the house today," change that thought to, "I am learning the new skills of mothering. This is the most important thing for me to be doing at this time." If you set high expectations for yourself each day and do not meet these goals, feelings of discouragement and despair often result. List-making and crossing off each task—no matter how basic—help some women to gain a sense of accomplishment. Table 4.1 may be of use to you during the first three to six weeks postpartum.

ACCEPTING HELP

"Mothering the mother" is often the best remedy for the baby blues. You need and deserve attention during this stressful time in your life. If you decide that you will graciously accept other people's help once the baby arrives, it will make your life a lot easier. Have some specific requests in mind when people offer their help: "A casserole would be wonderful," or "Could you take my two-year-old for a couple of hours?" Let friends and relatives know that you would welcome a home-cooked meal, babysitting, shopping, or cleaning services as a "baby gift."

Also, keep in mind that other people may not do things the same way you do. Instead of mentally complaining when "Aunt Barbara" washes the kitchen floor with the wrong detergent, relax, get back to your abdominal breathing, and use the time to sleep.

CRYING

During this time many women experience minor frustrations that could turn into major crying spells. Crying is one of the acceptable emotional releases that we have. If you feel like crying, experience the emotion fully by letting it out. You will feel much better afterwards. One of my students wrote, "The tears overwhelmed me in a big, forceful wave. . . . I didn't know why I was crying, because I felt so happy inside to have a healthy, beautiful baby boy. I cried for a short time and felt much better. It was a very unusual experience." Mood fluctuations are very common.

Table 4.1 Time Management		
Activity	**Time Spent**	**Comments**
Taking care of the baby	As much time as necessary	Believe in yourself and enjoy your new role.
Sleeping	As much time as possible	Sleep when the baby sleeps.
Being with your mate	As much time as possible	Have him share the care of the baby. Let him know what you need.
Personal hygiene	Shower or bathe once a day, more if necessary.	Keep the perineal area clean.
Cooking	Minimal time	Freeze meals in advance. Eat salads, fresh fruits, and easily made meals. Keep healthy snacks on hand.
Doing laundry	Minimal time	Wash baby clothes, diapers, blankets daily. Have husband or family help.
Cleaning house	Minimal time	Keep kitchens and bathrooms clean for health reasons. Ask for help!
Exercising	Try to work it into daily activities (while taking a shower or feeding the baby)	Do Abdominal Breaths (page 17), and continue doing the Squeeze (page 122) and stretches between feedings and while resting. Take walks with your baby.
Talking on phone	Limit calls from ten to fifteen minutes. Invest in an answering machine for those times when you are busy.	You should be resting!
Visits from family and friends	Limit visits from twenty to thirty minutes	Have visitors serve themselves. Use paper goods. Wear a robe so your company will know you're recuperating. (Yawning is a good way to hint that you need rest.)
Grocery shopping	Minimal time	Stock up on necessary items before the baby arrives. Try to have your husband or a friend do it until you feel up to it. It may then be a treat for you to go to the grocery store late in the evening—by yourself.

SOOTHING YOUR BABY WITH MUSIC

The *Baby Go To Sleep* audio cassette tape (page 312) can induce your newborn to sleep at an appropriate time. It contains classic lullabies such as "Hush, Little Baby," "Lullaby and Good Night," and "Rock-A-Bye Baby." These lullabies are sung in combination with the Peacemaker eucardial heartbeat. This tape actually induces sleep in every nine out of ten infants tested. To work most effectively, the *Baby Go To Sleep* tape should be played during the baby's first three months of life. Effective in calming over 91 percent of infant crying, this tape can give you much needed rest.

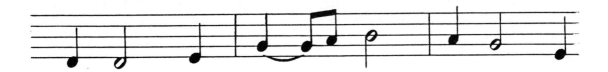

PATERNITY LEAVE

Fathers are often left out during the settling-in process because they are working. If possible, have your husband apply for a paternity leave (paid or unpaid). This will help him adjust to his new fatherhood role. He will also be able to help you at home and give you much needed emotional support.

TALK ABOUT HOW YOU FEEL

Discuss your feelings with your mate or with friends, especially if your birth experience wasn't what you wanted or planned for. Many Cesarean mothers resent their experience for years to come. If your experiences are too painful to talk about, you might try writing about them. Sometimes getting all your feelings down on paper is very therapeutic.

Five years ago, I was diagnosed with a rare neuromuscular disease called *myasthenia gravis*. This diagnosis was shortly followed by a series of strokes that left me unable to talk, read, and write. Quite a situation! Finding myself in a serious depression was one of a great number of effects. After I regained some of my lost faculties, I found that writing about my health battles helped me climb out of my depression and go forward with my life. If writing is not your style, try drawing your feelings. The method of your release is not important. What is important is that you do not lock your feelings inside thinking they will go away. Facing, accepting, and then talking, writing, or drawing a picture about your feelings will eventually make you feel better.

BABY BLUES OR POSTPARTUM DEPRESSION?

Many articles have been written on the "baby blues" and postpartum depression, and a variety of theories have been developed concerning the causes. The "blues" are considered different from the more serious postpartum depression. Baby blues usually begin early—between the third and fourteenth day after delivery. Symptoms—which include weepiness, anxious feelings, and subjective impairment of memory and concentration—appear and disappear without apparent cause. These symptoms usually last from twelve to twenty-four hours.

In medical circles, it is widely believed that the quick fluctuation in hormonal levels after the birth of the baby is the primary factor causing the blues. This is a physiological change that you will have to live through. A positive mental attitude can have a significant bearing on your experience. Following the guidelines in this chapter will help, too.

Sometimes the baby blues develop into postpartum depression, and this is more serious. Postpartum depression can be caused by hormonal imbalances; unrealistic expectations or "culture shock"; the resurfacing of unresolved issues such as unmet needs in childhood; or outside stressors such as new home, new job, new city, etc. The symptoms are probably the result of a combination of these factors.

These symptoms usually appear around the third week after delivery but may appear anytime during the first year. They may last for a few weeks or for a full year. The following symptoms are danger signals of which you should be aware:

- inability to cope with your new motherhood role
- a sense of powerlessness
- feelings of inadequacy
- feeling tired even after sleeping
- having bizarre thoughts
- impaired concentration or memory
- loss of normal interests
- headaches, numbness, chest pains, hyperventilating
- severe appetite changes
- extreme irritability leading to aggressive outbursts and total lack of control

If you experience one or any number of these symptoms during the postpartum period, you should seek professional help. Contact your obstetrician or midwife and get a referral to the correct person or agency, or you can contact the Hotline of Depression After Delivery, PO Box 1282, Morrisville, PA 19067, (215)295-3994 for help. There are local chapters that will assist you. Remember, it is a sign of strength, not weakness, to seek help.

POSTPARTUM GUIDELINES FOR COMBATTING THE "BLUES"

- Believe in yourself and in your capacities and instincts.
- Believe that you know your baby better than anyone else does.
- Believe that mothering is a learned rather than an instinctive role.
- Rest in bed whenever your baby sleeps.
- Don't feel guilty when napping.
- Eat a nourishing, well-balanced diet; drink plenty of water, juice, herbal tea, and milk.
- Keep your baby clean.
- Avoid strenuous work and heavy lifting for at least six weeks postpartum.
- Take some time each day just for yourself.

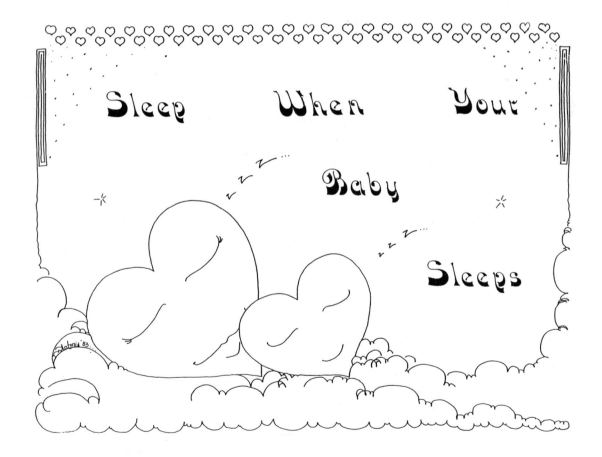

Make a copy of this page and post it on your refrigerator as a handy reminder!

CHAPTER FIVE
Postpartum Nutrition

"When can I go on a diet?" "What am I supposed to be eating to produce nutritionally sound milk?" "Why am I hungry or thirsty so often?" "Will I ever be able to close my jeans?" Sound familiar? These questions are the ones most commonly asked in Positive Parenting Fitness classes. Since basic information concerning a balanced, safe, and sound nutritional program is of vital importance to every new mother, this topic is usually discussed during the first session of Positive Parenting Fitness classes as well as in each succeeding class in the series.

Each body takes a different amount of time to regain its pregnancy shape. Following the nutritional and exercise guidelines in this book will help *your* body regain that shape while insuring your physical and mental well-being. Nutrition is especially important during the first six weeks after the baby arrives. This period should be one of nutritional build-up, but nutrition is often not the foremost concern of the new mother. Don't let this time of changes, erratic schedules, interrupted sleep, and great stresses; this time of exciting discovery and pleasure rob your body of the necessary nutrients.

YOUR IDEAL WEIGHT

Most new mothers lose about twenty pounds after giving birth. If you didn't gain twenty pounds during your pregnancy, you will, naturally, lose less. If you were overweight when you became pregnant and then gained twenty-five to thirty pounds, you will have to learn to eat lower-calorie, highly nutritious foods in order to reduce your new postpartum weight. Many nutritionalists calculate ideal weight according to height. The ideal weight for a woman who is five feet tall is 100 pounds. For every inch above five feet, another five pounds should be added for an ideal weight. Therefore, if you are five feet, three inches tall, your ideal weight should be 115 pounds. However, if your bone structure is large, you may find 120 pounds more comfortable for you. Once you have found your ideal weight, you should decide if you need to diet to reach that goal.

ADVICE FOR NURSING MOTHERS

Current research has indicated that a nursing mother of average weight and height—5 feet 3 inches to 5 feet 7 inches, weighing 115-145 pounds—needs approximately 2,500 calories a day to maintain her body weight as well as to produce enough milk for the baby. *This is only 500 calories more than the 2,000 calories that are required to maintain good health.*

If you are breastfeeding exclusively (or are producing 750 ccs of milk daily), and are consuming 500 extra calories daily, you should not gain weight as long as the diet you are eating is nutritionally balanced. If you think of the food that you eat as the ingredients for the nourishing milk that you are feeding your baby, you will be more inclined to make nutritious choices rather than consume empty calories or junk food.

Snacking

Many nursing mothers find that they become extremely thirsty and/or hungry as their baby is eating. I cannot remember any other time that I felt as thirsty as I did when nursing my two sons. It is a good idea for the nursing mother to have a glass of liquid handy while the baby is drinking. Keep iced water or iced unsugared herbal teas on hand at all times so you can easily drink something before and while you nurse. Be careful about drinking most fruit juices because they are calorie-laden. If fruit juice is what you prefer or all that you have on hand, mix a half glass of juice with a half glass of water to cut down on calories.

The hunger pangs can be startling as well. You may have experienced the same deep feeling of hunger when you were pregnant. Eating four to six small meals a day will keep up your energy level; with so little sleep this will really help. The snacks suggested at the conclusion of this section were developed with concern for high nutrition and a low calorie count.

If you are nursing, do not drastically restrict your calories. Choose your diet and snacks more carefully instead. In many cases, the foods with the highest caloric content, such as potato chips, candy, and donuts, are very low in nutritional value. By balancing and choosing foods carefully, you can regain your prepregnancy shape.

POSTPARTUM WEIGHT LOSS

After your six-week check-up, it may be wise to discuss your diet plans with your caregiver. Some caregivers may want you to have "established" sleeping patterns before dieting. The weight-loss diet that begins on page 62 should only be utilized *after* the first six weeks postpartum. Your body needs full caloric nourishment during the first six weeks to replace depleted stores of iron and other essential vitamins and minerals that were used by your baby.

Weight Loss For Breastfeeding Mothers

There have been some recent findings concerning weight loss for breastfeeding mothers. Some studies show that if you lose weight too quickly, fat-soluble toxins are released from the body's fat stores through breast milk. If you've worked in areas with dangerous materials, such as pesticides or chemicals, you may be a victim. The average person working in a safe, clean environment shouldn't worry. However, more studies are in progress. If you are nursing or bottle-feeding, you have to make a personal decision about weight loss. Use common sense if you want to diet while you are nursing. If your baby shows no sign of hunger and grows at a proper rate and your breasts remain full, you can afford to limit calories.

GENERAL GUIDELINES FOR WEIGHT-LOSS PROGRAMS

- Before starting *any* diet, discuss your plans for weight-reduction with your caregiver.
- Begin with a well-established nursing relationship with your baby. Allow at least two to three weeks postpartum to achieve this relationship.
- Start your weight-loss diet no sooner than six weeks postpartum.
- Begin to observe the things you eat; notice the foods that contain empty calories, such as donuts, cookies, chips, and candy. These low-nutrition foods provide nothing more than fat and sugar calories.
- Eliminate empty calories from your diet.
- Reduce your caloric intake to 2,200 calories per day, 500 of which will go to feed your baby. Non-nursing mothers should reduce their daily caloric intake to 1,800.
- Your average weight loss should be between 1 1/2 -2 pounds per week. If you lose weight slowly, it will stay off.
- Make every calorie count with highly nutritious foods. Eat foods high in iron (liver, whole grains, potatoes, green leafy vegetables) and zinc (oysters, herring, liver, eggs). Increasing fiber in your diet (raw vegetables and fruits) will provide more bulk without adding calories and will satisfy your appetite.
- You should supplement your daily diet with 30 milligrams of iron, 500 milligrams of calcium, and a good multiple vitamin or one of your prenatal vitamins. Be aware that an iron supplement might cause constipation.

A BALANCED APPROACH TO FOOD

To achieve harmony and balance in your diet, you must first have a positive mental attitude about the food that is eaten. Secondly, have a well understood nutritional program; finally, eat foods in a state that is as close to natural as possible.

In order to keep your body centered and productive as it heals following the birth of a baby, you must follow a pattern of balanced and nutritious eating. A simple way to understand the components of a balanced diet is to think of four main food groups:

• **Protein**: meat, meatless, and complementary proteins (meat, fish, poultry, eggs, dried beans, nuts, nut butters, and seeds)
• **Calcium**: milk, yogurt, cheese, sardines (with bones), sesame seeds, and vegetables such as kale and broccoli
• **Whole grains and starchy vegetables**: breads, pastas, potatoes, sweet potatoes, and winter squash
• **Fruits and vegetables**: fresh, dried, and the juice from those with Vitamin C (oranges, tangerines, cauliflower) and those with Vitamin A (cantaloupe, peaches, carrots, leafy greens)

Most of your dietary selections should come from these groups. A small percentage of your diet—500 calories per week—may come from a fifth group of "luxury calories." Remember, it is this fifth group that will keep those extra pounds on your hips and thighs.

• **Luxury foods**: butter, vegetable oils, salad dressings, candy, cookies, cakes, donuts, pastry, gravies, chips, French fries.

POSITIVE PARENTING FITNESS SAFE REDUCING DIET

Table 5.1 provides a general outline of the Safe Reducing Diet. Serving sizes of specific foods can be found in Tables 5.2 through 5.7.

Protein

Protein is one of the most important elements in growth and development. It is the building block for muscles, blood, antibodies, enzymes, hormones, skin, hair, nails, all internal organs, and the formation of milk during lactation.

Protein is supplied by both animal and vegetable sources. If meat is a major source of protein in your diet, you can keep the percentage of fat at an acceptable level by eating only extra-lean beef, lamb, and pork, which are excellent sources of iron and B vitamins.

Table 5.1   Guidelines for the Safe Reducing Diet

Calorie Source	Daily Servings for Breastfeeding Women	Daily Servings for Non-Breastfeeding Women
Complete protein (meat, meatless, or complementary)	2-3	2-3
Calcium	5	4
Whole grains and starchy vegetables	5	3
Fruits and vegetables with Vitamin C with Vitamin A	1 1	1 1
Leafy green vegetables	2 (1 tossed salad = 1 serving)	2
Fats (butter, margarine, vegetable oil)	3-6 teaspoons or less	3-6 teaspoons or less
Liquids (water, juices, herbal teas, milk)	8-12	6-8

In addition, up to 500 luxury calories (page 72) may be consumed each week.

*This weight-loss diet was developed and tested by Jacquie Burzycki, RN, Positive Parenting Fitness Master Teacher and instructor of Positive Parenting Fitness classes at the Norwich YMCA in Norwich, Connecticut. She and her students used this diet for permanent weight reduction through gradual weight loss. It is based on *Exchange List for Meal Planning* (American Diabetes Association, 1986), the *Weight Watchers Quick-Success Program* (1987), *Nutrition Almanac* (Nutrition Search, Inc., 1979), *The Very Important Pregnancy Program* by Gail Brewer (Emmanus, PA: Rodale Press, 1988), and *A Successful Nursing Diet* by Myron Winick, MD (*Mothers Today*, Jan.-Feb., 1985).

Increase your intake of lower-fat animal protein such as chicken (no skin), turkey (no skin), veal, and white, flaky fish. Limit your intake of processed meats such as bacon, salami, bologna, and other luncheon meats. These foods contain nitrites, nitrates, and other additives that have been shown to cause stomach cancer in rats. These meats also have built-in fat, which won't help your weight-loss plans. Prepare meats by trimming all visible fat and by removing any skin. Broil, bake, or steam meats. *Do not fry foods*, for the added fats will go directly to your hips!

Protein is either complete or incomplete depending on the number of essential amino acids it contains. Complete protein foods (all animal products and by-products) contain these essential amino acids in the proper proportion to meet your body's requirement. Incomplete protein foods (legumes, grains, seeds, nuts, etc.) are missing one or more essential amino acids. By serving the incomplete protein—cereal—with a complete protein—milk—or by serving two complementary incomplete proteins—peanut butter with whole-wheat bread, or beans with corn—you will have all the essential amino acids. (A very good resource on protein is *Diet for a Small Planet* by Francis Lappe Moore.)

Recommended Sources of Protein

Eat two to three servings per day of the low-fat, protein-rich foods found in Table 5.2. (Four ounces of uncooked meat weighs approximately three ounces when cooked.)

Calcium

Calcium is the most abundant mineral in the body; it is a basic component of bones and teeth, which are 99 percent calcium. In addition to forming strong bones and teeth,

Table 5.2   Protein: Daily Serving Suggestions

Food	Serving Size
Fish—fresh or frozen fish or shellfish, canned fish (drained well)	3 ounces
Poultry—chicken, turkey, cornish hens, pheasant (skin removed)	3 ounces
Veal—leg, loin, rib, shank, shoulder, cutlets	3 ounces
Cottage cheese, pot cheese	1/3 cup
Beans, lentils, peas	3/4 ounce (dry) 2 ounces (cooked)
Tofu	3 ounces
Peanut butter (omit 1 fat serving)	1 tablespoon
Eggs	1 medium
Egg substitute	1/4 cup

No more than 16 ounces of your total weekly protein intake should come from the following high-fat, protein-rich foods:

Beef	3 ounces
Lamb	3 ounces
Pork	3 ounces

calcium is necessary for the formation of healthy blood and for the regulation of heart rate, muscle growth, and contractions. Calcium is essential to various functions of the nervous system and can also ease insomnia.

Milk is a leading source of calcium. Milk is also a source of phosphorous, magnesium, protein, Vitamin B$_{12}$, folacin, and Vitamins A and D. Some of these vitamins and minerals are needed for calcium to function properly. A number of adults and children are, however, unable to digest dairy products due to reduced levels of *lactase,* an enzyme that breaks down *lactose* (the sugar in milk).

Symptoms of lactose intolerance include gastric disturbances such as indigestion, gas, diarrhea, or constipation in adults, and sometimes colic in infants. In such cases, yogurt with active cultures that don't have large amounts of milk solids added, and lactose-reduced milk are sometimes tolerated. In other cases, abstinence from all dairy products is necessary. If you are intolerant of calcium foods, consult your caregiver for an adequate calcium supplement. Lactating women may replace four milk servings with two additional breads (see page 67) and two additional proteins (see page 64)for caloric purposes. Non-lactating women may replace two milk servings with one additional bread and one additional protein.

Recommended Sources of Calcium

Nursing mothers should have five servings of the following low-fat dairy products found in Table 5.3 each day; non-nursing mothers should have four daily servings. Each serving provides approximately 12 grams of carbohydrates, 9 grams of protein, trace amounts of fat, and approximately 90 calories. (One cup is equal to eight ounces.)

Carbohydrates

Carbohydrates are needed to produce the energy for all body functions. Whole grains and cereals, and dried beans and peas are also good sources of iron and B-complex vitamins, which provide energy and help stabilize mood swings.

Recommended Sources of Carbohydrates

Nursing mothers should eat five servings of the following grains and starchy vegetables found in Table 5.4 each day. Non-nursing mothers should have three daily servings. Each portion provides approximately 15 grams of carbohydrates, 2 grams of protein, and 68 calories.

Table 5.3   Calcium: Daily Serving Suggestions

Food	Serving Size 1 cup = 8 ounces
Skim or non-fat milk	1 cup
Powdered (non-fat dry, before adding liquid)	1/3 cup
Canned, evaporated skim milk	1/2 cup
Buttermilk made from skim milk	1 cup
Yogurt made from skim milk (plain, unflavored)	1 cup
Soymilk products (90 calories per 8-ounce serving)	1 cup

The following dairy products are higher in fat and should be limited to occasional use:

Food		Serving Size
Low-fat (1 percent) milk	(add 20 luxury calories)	1 cup
Low-fat (2 percent) milk	(add 40 luxury calories)	1 cup
Whole milk	(add 60 luxury calories)	1 cup
Canned, evaporated whole milk	(add 60 luxury calories)	1 cup
Buttermilk made from whole milk	(add 60 luxury calories)	1 cup
Yogurt (plain) from whole milk	(add 60 luxury calories)	1 cup

Other calcium sources include shellfish, eggs, sardines (with bones), salmon, leafy green vegetables, broccoli, and kale. Three tablespoons of sesame seeds provide as much calcium as in one cup of milk.

Vegetables

The generous use of vegetables will contribute to your good health. Vegetables are excellent sources of Vitamin A and Vitamin C. Vitamin A is a vital component in the growth and repair of tissues, including your skin. It also helps protect the mucous membranes, which prevent the invasion of disease-causing organisms. Vitamin A aids in the digestion of proteins and in the formation of strong teeth, rich blood, and good eyesight. Dark green and deep yellow vegetables are particularly good sources of Vitamin A. Green leafy vegetables are also a good source of calcium. Since vegetables are also very low in calories and fat, they are excellent choices to include in a weight-loss diet.

Fresh vegetables should always be your first choice. The vitamins present in vegetables are perishable and easily destroyed by heat, light, and soaking. The best method of preparation is to steam your vegetables in a vegetable steamer. Frozen vegetables are your second choice when fresh are not available. Canned vegetables should be your last choice.

Table 5.4   Carbohydrates: Daily Serving Suggestions

Foods	Serving Size
Breads and Starchy Vegetables	
Arrowroot crackers	3
Bagel (small)	1/2 (1 ounce)
Bread (any type)	1 slice
Bread (reduced calorie or cocktail)	2 slices
Bread crumbs	3 tablespoons
Breadsticks	1 (3/4 ounce)
Butter cracker	5
Corn	1/3 cup
Corn on the cob	1 small (4" long)
English muffin	1/2 (1 ounce)
Frankfurter roll	1/2 (1 ounce)
Frankfurter roll (reduced calorie)	1 (1 ounce)
Graham cracker (2 1/2" square)	2
Hamburger roll	1/2
Lima beans	1/2 cup
Matzo (4" x 6")	1/2
Melba toast (round)	6
Melba toast (slices)	4
Oyster crackers	20
Parsnips	2/3 cup
Peas	1/2 cup
Pita bread (3" round)	1 (1 ounce)
Potato, mashed	1/2 cup
Potato, white (small)	1
Pretzels (3 1/8" long x 1/8" diameter)	25
Pumpkin	3/4 cup
Roll (plain)	1 (1 ounce)
Saltines	6
Soda crackers	4
Tortilla (6" round)	1
Winter squash, acorn or butternut	1/2
Yam or sweet potato	1/4 cup
Grains	
Cereal (cold, unsweetened)	1/2 cup
Cereal (cooked)	1/2 cup
Cornmeal (dry)	2 tablespoons
Flour	3 tablespoons
Pasta (cooked)	1/2 cup
Popcorn (air popped, no butter, large kernel)	3 cups
Rice (cooked)	1/2 cup
Rice cakes	2
Wheat germ	1/4 cup

Table 5.4 – *"Continued"*

Foods	Serving Size
Prepared Foods (omit 1 additional fat)	
Biscuit (2" diameter)	1
Corn bread (2" x 2" x 1")	1
Corn muffin (2 " diameter)	1
French fried potatoes (3 1/2" long)	8
Pancakes (5" diameter)	1
Waffles (5" diameter)	1

Recommended Vegetables

Eat at least two servings of green leafy vegetables and one serving of deep yellow/orange vegetables each day. Each 1/2-cup serving provides approximately 5 grams of carbohydrates, 2 grams of protein, and 25 calories.

Nutritious Vegetables

Beet greens
Chards
Chinese cabbage
Collards
Dandelion greens
Dark green varieties of
  lettuce (romaine, Boston,
  chickory, escarole)
Kale
Mustard greens
Parsley
Spinach
Turnip greens

Lower-Nutrient Vegetables

Mushrooms
Okra
Onions
Radishes
Rhubarb
Rhutabaga
Sauerkraut
String beans (yellow or green)
Summer squash
Tomatoes
Zucchini

Gas-Producing Vegetables

Asparagus
Bean sprouts
Beets
Broccoli
Cabbage
Carrots
Cauliflower
Celery
Cucumbers or dill pickles
Eggplant
Green peppers

Fruits

Some fruits are rich in vitamins: Vitamin C is abundant in citrus fruits, raspberries, strawberries, mangoes, cantaloupes, nectarines, and peaches. Fruits that are high in potassium include bananas and apricots, while yellow fruits are high in folacin.

Vitamin C is particularly important as it is used to maintain collagen (connective tissue), which is the protein necessary for the formation of skin, ligaments, and bones. Vitamin C is also needed for the healing of wounds and for the prevention of hemorrhages. It fights bacterial infections and reduces the effects of some allergy-producing substances on the body.

Fruits are best when served fresh; fresh fruit served in the height of its season is the most nutritious and delicious. Dried fruits should be your second choice. Frozen fruits follow as the next choice, while canned fruit, no sugar added, can be used as a last choice.

Recommended Fruits

Eat at least one serving of yellow fruit each day. Each of the following fruit servings found in Table 5.5 provides approximately 10 grams of carbohydrates and 40 calories.

Fats

Fats are an essential part of good nutrition; they provide the most concentrated source of energy in our diet. Fats also act as carriers for the fat-soluble vitamins (A,D,E, and K) to the body tissue. Fats protect the internal organs by surrounding them with fatty deposits; they prolong digestion by slowing down the release of gastric juices into the stomach. Fats can, therefore, contribute to a feeling of fullness after a meal.

There are two types of fat: saturated and unsaturated. Saturated fats are those that harden at room temperature. Saturated fats come primarily from animal sources, with the exception of coconut oil and palm kernel oil. Unsaturated fats (mono- and polyunsaturated) remain liquid at room temperature and are derived from the vegetable kingdom. Some vegetable shortenings as well as margarine have undergone hydrogenation, thereby creating a more saturated form of fat.

The average American consumes far more fat than is necessary to carry out normal body processes. This abnormal amount of fat is a major contributing factor to high rates of obesity, heart disease, and cancer. Fat is one component in our diet that if reduced will generate weight loss while promoting good health. Reducing the fat in your diet will help you establish good eating habits, which will, in turn, be passed on to your child.

Table 5.5   Fruits: Daily Serving Suggestions

Food	Serving Size
Apple juice	1/3 cup
Apples	1 small
Applesauce	1/2 cup
Apricots, dried	4 halves
Apricots, fresh	2 medium
Bananas	1/2 small
Cherries	10 large
Cranberries (no sugar)	as desired
Cranberry juice (low cal)	1 cup
Dates	2
Figs	1
Grape juice	1/4 cup
Grapefruit	1/2
Grapefruit juice	1/2 cup
Grapes	12
Kiwi	1 medium
Mangoes	1/4 small
Melons:	
cantaloupe	1/4 small
honeydew	1/8 medium
watermelon	1 cup
Nectarines	1 small
Orange juice	1/2 cup
Oranges	1 small
Papaya	3/4 cup
Peaches	1 medium
Persimmons	1 medium
Pineapple juice	1/3 cup
Pineapples	1/2 cup
Plums	2 medium
Prune juice	1/2 cup
Prunes	2 medium
Raisins	2 tablespoons
Strawberries	1 cup
Tangerines	1 medium

Recommended Sources of Fat

Fat consumption should be 25 to 30 percent of your total caloric intake, or from 3 to 6 teaspoons per day. Foods high in polyunsaturated fats—the most desirable kind of fats—are shown in boldface print in Table 5.6. Each portion provides approximately 5 grams of fat and 45 calories. (Measure each portion carefully to insure sufficient consumption of these concentrated energy calories.)

Table 5.6   Fats: Serving Amounts

Food	Portion
Avocado (4"diameter)	1/8
Bacon, crisp	1 strip
Butter	1 teaspoon
Cream, heavy	1 tablespoon
Cream, light or sour	2 tablespoons
Lard	1 teaspoon
Margarine, soft, tub or stick	1 teaspoon
Mayonnaise (made with corn, cottonseed, safflower, soy or sunflower oil)	1 teaspoon
Nuts	
Almonds	10
Peanuts	
Spanish	20
Virginia	10
Pecans (large)	2
Walnuts (small)	5
Other (small)	6
Oil (corn, cottonseed, safflower, soy, sunflower, olive, peanut)	1 teaspoon
Olives (small)	5 small
Salad Dressings	
French or Italian	1 tablespoon
Mayonnaise type	2 teaspoons
Salt pork	3/4 cube

Luxury Calories

No more than 500 calories per week should come from the luxury calories found in Table 5.7. Luxury calories will add variety and zest to your food, which will help you to stay on your weight-loss diet. Don't deprive yourself of these little extras.

NUTRITIONAL PITFALLS TO AVOID

A Lack of Vitamins and Minerals

During the last trimester of pregnancy, your body developed stores of minerals that were passed on to your baby. During the postpartum period, you need to replenish these depleted stores of vital substances. Therefore, *continue taking your prenatal vitamins as well as an iron supplement for at least two to three months postpartum.* You should be taking thirty

Table 5.7   Luxury Calories

Food	Serving Size
5-10-Calorie Foods	
Cheese, hard grated	1 teaspoon
Cocoa, unsweetened	2 teaspoons
Coconut, shredded	1 teaspoon
Cornstarch or flour	1 teaspoon
Creamer, non-dairy	1 teaspoon
Egg white (hard-boiled)	1/2 egg
Honey, sugar, syrup	1/2 teaspoon
Ketchup	2 teaspoons
Relish, any type	1 teaspoon
Seeds	1/2 teaspoon
50-Calorie Foods	
Cream, any type	1 tablespoon
Half-and-half	2 tablespoons
Jams, jellies, preserves	1 tablespoon
Sauce: barbecue, chili, seafood, cocktail, steak	3 tablespoons
Tartar sauce	2 tablespoons
Tomato purée or sauce	1/2 cup
Whipped topping	1/4 cup
100-Calorie Foods	
Beer	8 fluid ounces
Beer, light	12 fluid ounces
Butter	1 tablespoon
Butter, whipped	2 tablespoons
Coleslaw	1/2 cup
Cream cheese	2 tablespoons
Cream cheese, whipped	3 tablespoons
Gelatin, fruit-flavored	1/2 cup

to sixty milligrams of iron daily in either supplement form or by eating iron-rich foods such as liver, legumes, whole grains, eggs, leafy greens, oysters (from safe, certified harvesting areas) and other shellfish, blackstrap molasses, seaweed, nuts, and cherries. (Legumes, leafy greens, and blackstrap molasses are gas-producing and should be avoided if gas is a problem.) Remember that taking vitamin pills is not a substitute for good nutrition but contributes to the total workings and health of the body.

Breastfeeding women should talk to their pediatricians about a daily Vitamin-D supplement to be given directly to their babies, because breast milk does not contain adequate amounts of this vitamin. Also worthy of discussion is a daily supplement of fluoride for the baby. You have to discuss the amount and need for this supplement with your doctor, for it depends on how much fluoride is contained in your community's water supply and in baby foods. Do not self-prescribe fluoride or Vitamin D. Check with your caregiver.

Alcohol

Sometimes the frustrations of new parenthood will get to you. Some health-care providers feel that an occasional glass of wine(no more than three ounces) or an eight-ounce glass of beer can help you relax. Some also think that it helps your "let-down reflex" in which the act of nursing stimulates the sinuses and ducts in the breasts to fill with milk. However, drinking alcohol will not solve any of your problems. Alcohol will reduce your levels of water-soluble vitamins, such as Vitamin B_1, B_2, B_6, B_{12}, C, niacin, pantothenic acid, and folacin. Talking about your life with all of its frustrations in a Positive Parenting Fitness class or any other new-mother support group will benefit you much, much more.

Caffeine

Coffee, regular teas, most colas and other sodas, cocoa, chocolate, and many prescription and non-prescription drugs contain caffeine, which is a chemical stimulant. Some studies have shown birth defects in rats that were fed exceedingly high amounts of caffeine. Most experts agree that there is no evidence to show that moderate amounts of caffeine (two cups a day) will harm your baby in utero. Approximately 1 percent of the caffeine that a nursing mother drinks appears in her breast milk within fifteen minutes. Therefore, it makes the most sense to drink caffeinated liquids after you nurse. Try brewing coffee by combining half the amount of regular coffee with half decaffeinated. Coffee and tea make no significant contribution to your diet, but they may be pleasurable choices. If you decide to cut back on caffeine or cut it out completely, you will not be compromising your nutrition. You may actually be improving it. Be aware—especially if you are breastfeeding—that coffee and regular tea contain organic acids that can bind with some minerals such as iron, magnesium, zinc, and calcium. Therefore, your body can't absorb these minerals.

Smoking

If you decide to continue smoking, try not to smoke while feeding your baby. Try not to be near the baby when you are smoking. Research has shown that babies exposed to secondary smoke in their environment are more prone to bronchial illnesses. Although new motherhood is a very stressful time, it might be a good time to cut down on your use of cigarettes. If you continue to smoke, be aware that smokers need more Vitamin C in their diet.

PRACTICAL HINTS FOR WEIGHT-CONSCIOUS MOTHERS

- Try to eat while sitting down at the table.
- Chew your food well, even though your time for eating may be limited. Don't gulp down what you eat.
- Take a few minutes for eating and enjoying your food. Do not read, watch television, or do other things when you are eating.
- Eat four to six small meals a day to keep your energy level high.
- Eat only when you are truly hungry. Keep track of what you eat each day.
- Drink plenty of water, herbal teas, unsweetened fruit juices, and milk. Avoid calorie-laden soda. Try a *Fruity Milkshake* instead (recipe on page 86).
- When you are in the mood for something sweet, reach for a piece of fruit. A medium-sized orange is only 75 calories, while a regular-sized Hershey bar is 300!
- Limit the amount of oil in your diet to three to six teaspoons a day. Remember that many foods already have built-in fat. The recipe for *Better Butter* (page 85) has only 38 calories per teaspoon, while regular butter has 100.
- Use bean sprouts on sandwiches and in salads for added crispness, vitamins, and minerals. See the inset Making a Bean Sprouter, page 83.
- Whenever possible, try substituting small amounts of mustard such as Dijon, which is low in calories, for mayonnaise, which is high in calories.
- Take the amount of food that you plan to eat from its package, and then put the package away (and out of sight).
- Take the baby out for a one or two-mile walk each day. A walk provides fresh air and a change of scenery for both you and your baby. And walking burns calories.
- Share some play time each day with your baby as you practice your Positive Parenting Fitness exercises and breathing. Deep breathing burns calories and helps you relax.
- Have patience with your body. Let it slowly regain its shape through good eating habits, regular exercise, and a bit of faith. When you feel "yucky" about your body, practice the Moon Salute (page 159) for five minutes.
- Crash diets are not beneficial to you or your baby. Usually the weight lost on these types

of diets is gained back quickly because you haven't changed your eating patterns. During a crash diet your body learns to burn less calories when it gets less. When you go back to eating normally, your body stores every calorie it doesn't burn as fat.

• If you cannot seem to lose weight, you might consider joining a support group such as Weight Watchers. You can contact the nutrition department of your local hospital for support-group information.

HINTS FOR QUICK, HEALTHFUL MEALS AND SNACKS

New mothers are often surprised to find that there is very limited time for food preparation and eating once the baby arrives. Often, if they find time to prepare a well-balanced and tasty meal, the baby will be fussy while they are trying to eat it. There are some short cuts, which some of my students have discovered, that may be helpful to you.

1. When preparing a recipe that freezes well, double it and freeze a second portion for a future meal.
2. Make an extra-large salad with a variety of leafy greens and other vegetables such as lettuce, celery, cabbage, raw broccoli and cauliflower, Chinese cabbage, carrots, green and red peppers, cooked beets, zucchini, raw yellow squash, and radishes. After washing the vegetables, dry them carefully and place them in an airtight plastic container. If you do not add any dressing, this salad will keep well for three days. The vitamin content will diminish slightly, but being able to reach for a bowl of salad is more beneficial than grabbing a cupcake. Try a reduced-calorie, buttermilk dressing for a nutritional boost. (Cabbage, cauliflower, green peppers, and leafy greens are gas-producing and should be eaten in moderation, or avoided completely if necessary.)
3. Try preparing dishes that take very little time to cook such as *Sylvia's Almond Chow Mein* (page 82).
4. In a bowl of cold water, keep an assortment of raw, cut vegetables. Celery and carrot sticks, string beans, and pepper rings are just a few vegetables to use for these quick, crunchy snacks.
5. Cooking your "veggies" with a steamer will save time and insure more vitamins in your food. Steam until the vegetables are brightly colored.
6. An open-faced grilled sandwich is a great idea for a quick meal. Using whole wheat or any other whole grain bread, create an open-faced sandwich with meat loaf, tuna fish, turkey slices, etc. Place some grated cheese, such as cheddar, mozzarella, or Monterey Jack on top and grill for a few minutes under the broiler or in the microwave. Serve with a salad for a quick, satisfying meal.
7. Keep whole wheat pita bread handy and fill it with leftover meats, vegetables, and cheese. Heat or eat as is.

Postpartum Nutrition: An Overview

•Try to eat foods that are in a state as close to natural as possible.

•Eat four to six small meals a day.

•If you are breastfeeding, don't take any oral contraceptives for at least six weeks postpartum. These pills will diminish the amount of milk that you produce.

•Do not take any kind of antihistamines; they will reduce your milk production.

•Do not take any laxatives, barbiturates, or other drugs during the lactation period; they will be transmitted through your milk to your baby.

•Keep your alcohol consumption to a minimum; the alcohol will be passed to the baby through your breast milk in very concentrated amounts.

•If you continue to smoke, try to do it away from your baby. Remember that you are polluting your new baby's lungs with cigarette smoke that you release into the air. Change your shirt for each cigarette smoked, for the smoke sticks to it.

•If you are nursing, increase your daily fluid intake to eight to twelve glasses of liquid a day to provide liquid volume for breast milk and for your production of urine.

•Eat only when you are truly hungry and choose foods wisely.

•If you indulge in an occasional candy bar or donut, do not let a guilty wave engulf you. Next time, try a *Quick Energy Snack* (recipe on page 87), which is for those times when you want a sweet, natural, quick energy boost. The calorie content of this recipe is very high, so don't eat more than three to four small pieces. The total caloric content of this recipe is 1,750 calories. Cut into twenty-four small pieces, each piece contains 73 calories. Eat it sparingly, but enjoy it fully. It contains many more vitamins, minerals, and nutrients than a candy bar and is a very good natural substitute.

•If your baby is up and alert at dinner time, put him on the table in an infant seat so he can interact with you and your mate. Babies are very social beings and will benefit from your company and stimulation.

•Since each woman experiences different reactions during the postpartum period, the advice within this chapter may be helpful to you. Or you may find other practical solutions. The guiding principles in the postpartum period are moderation and common sense as you adjust and begin to enjoy your new life.

SAMPLE MENUS

Miriam Erick, author of *D.I.E.T. for Pregnancy* and registered dietitian at Brigham and Women's Hospital, Boston, MA, has developed suggested menus that will help you utilize the Positive Parenting Fitness diet (summarized in Table 5.1) more easily. The recipes have been created with ease of preparation in mind for the busy postpartum woman. The following sample menus introduce colorful and appealing meals while offering a new approach to standard food. Recipes featured in the menus can be found in the recipe section beginning on page 79.

MENU ONE

Breakfast

2 slices French toast
1/2 cup mandarin orange slices,
topped with sprig of fresh mint

Carbohydrates	Protein	Fat	Calories
54 grams	13 grams	5 grams	348
		(10 grams of fat if margarine used)	

Lunch

1 cup *Potato Cheesy Soup* (page 84)
Salad of dark lettuce greens, 1/2 tomato,
cucumber slices, and 1 tablespoon buttermilk dressing

Carbohydrates	Protein	Fat	Calories
29 grams	17 grams	13 grams	305

Dinner

1 cup *Stir-Fried Beef* (page 84)
3/4 cup plain boiled rice
1/2 cup ice milk topped with 1/4 cup fresh strawberries

Carbohydrates	Protein	Fat	Calories
61 grams	46 grams	20 grams	610

Snack

8 ounces tomato juice
3 celery sticks

Carbohydrates	Protein	Fat	Calories
17 grams	1 gram	1 gram	75

MENU TWO

Breakfast

3/4 cup English oatmeal (prepared with 1 cup skim milk)*
topped with 1 small nectarine, chopped

Carbohydrates	Protein	Fat	Calories
44 grams	10 grams	2 grams	235

Lunch

1/2 medium cantaloupe
filled with 1/2 cup low-fat cottage cheese,
and topped with 1/4 cup blueberries
1 small crunchy French bread roll with 1 pat margarine

Carbohydrates	Protein	Fat	Calories
44 grams	17 grams	10 grams	326

Dinner

Small chicken breast (3 1/2 ounces with no skin), baked
1 medium baked potato
1/2 cup beets
1/2 cup broccoli spears
1 cup skim milk
1 baked apple with 1 tablespoon raisins

Carbohydrates	Protein	Fat	Calories
69 grams	36 grams	25 grams	645

Snack

1 slice raisin toast topped with
1 tablespoon skim milk ricotta cheese

Carbohydrates	Protein	Fat	Calories
19 grams	4 grams	1 gram	100

*When cooking oatmeal, prepare at least six servings at one time. Eat your breakfast serving and refrigerate the rest. Oatmeal microwaves wonderfully, saving you time and pot-washing for the rest of the week. Better nutrition for less money!

RECIPES

Herbal Recipes

According to herbalist Jeannine Parvati Baker in *Hygieia: A Woman's Herbal,* iron tea and calcium tea are two examples of good, basic teas that replace needed minerals and fluids for nursing mothers. These teas are a source of extra energy and a feeling of peacefulness.

Iron-Rich Tea

Equal parts of:
Beet powder, dried
Dandelion root, dried
Dulse, dried
Nettle, dried
Parsley, dried
Yellow dock, dried

Mix dried herbs together thoroughly. Put 1-2 teaspoons of the dried herb mixture in a cup. Add 1 cup of boiling water. Steep 35-40 minutes.

Calcium-Rich Tea

Equal parts of:
Borage, dried
Chamomile, dried
Comfrey, dried
Oat straw, dried

Mix dried herbs together thoroughly. Put 1 teaspoon of the dried herb mixture in a cup. Add 1 cup of boiling water. Steep 35-40 minutes.

Susun S. Weed, in her book *Wise Woman Herbal for the Childbearing Year,* recommends the following teas to help you deal with postpartum depression and to improve your breastfeeding. She points out that licorice favorably affects the hormonal balance and cheers the spirit; however, a word of caution is offered by Miriam Erick, RD, who warns that licorice should be used with caution by people with hypertension.

Ms. Weed also says that raspberry leaves help tone the uterus and ovaries and help increase the body's available calcium, making life seem easier. Rosemary increases the milk flow, adds calcium, tones the liver, and is the *Wise Woman* favorite for depression. Skullcap is also a source of calcium and is a superb nerve strengthener and soother; prolonged use promotes emotional calm. Drink two or more cups daily for several weeks up to two months.

Postpartum Depression Brew

1/2 ounce licorice root, dried
1 ounce raspberry leaves, dried
1 ounce rosemary leaves, dried
1 ounce skullcap, dried

Crush the dried herbs and mix them together thoroughly. Put 2 teaspoons of the dried herb mixture in a cup. Add 1 cup boiling water. Steep.

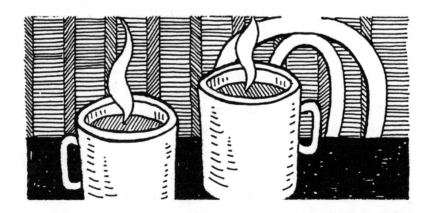

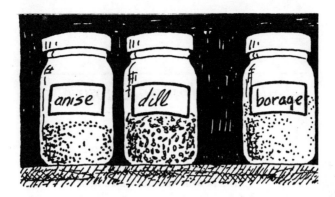

Blessed thistle (borage) stimulates the milk to flow and helps restore vitality to weary mothers. Raspberry and nettle supply vitamins and minerals, notably calcium, which is needed for plentiful lactation. The aromatic seeds increase milk production and tone the digestive system; their powers are carried through the breast milk and into your nursing child, curtailing colic and indigestion. This brew may be drunk freely, up to two quarts a day.

Nursing Formula

---

1 ounce blessed thistle (borage) leaves, dried
1 ounce raspberry or nettle leaves, dried
1 teaspoon of any of the following seeds:
anise, caraway, coriander, cumin, dill, fennel

Yield: 1/2 gallon

Place leaves in a half-gallon jar and fill to the top with boiling water. Cap tightly and let steep overnight. Strain out herbs and refrigerate liquid until needed.

As you prepare to nurse, pour off one cupful of the brew and heat it nearly to a boil. Pour it over 1 teaspoonful of the desired aromatic seeds. Cool for five minutes before drinking.

Main Dishes

Sylvia's Almond Chow Mein

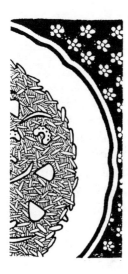

2 tablespoons vegetable oil
1-2 cloves garlic, minced
1/2 pound spinach, shredded
3-4 large bok choy leaves, shredded
1 onion, sliced
3-4 stalks celery, sliced
1 red pepper, diced
1 green pepper, diced
6-8 water chestnuts, diced
1 cup almonds, chopped
1/2 cup sunflower seeds
1/2 cup pumpkin seeds, chopped
3/4 cup vegetable broth
1/3 cup cold water
2 tablespoons cornstarch or arrowroot
2-3 tablespoons tamari soy sauce

Serves: 4

Heat the oil in a large frying pan or wok. Add the garlic and stir until golden brown (be careful not to burn). Add all of the vegetables, nuts, and seeds. Stir until coated with oil and cook until the onion begins to look transparent. Add the vegetable broth and cover. Simmer for 3-4 minutes.

While the vegetables are simmering, mix together the water, cornstarch or arrowroot, and tamari soy sauce in a small bowl. Add this mixture to the wok, stirring constantly until it forms a thick gravy. Be careful not to overcook—the vegetables should be bright in color when serving.

This chow mein is delicious when served over hot brown rice or any other cooked grain. For variety, other vegetables and leftover meat, fish, or chicken can be used.

French Toast

4 slices bread
1 egg
1 1/2 cups low-fat milk
Cinnamon
Small pat margarine (optional)

Mix egg and milk thoroughly. Dip bread in mixture, coating both sides. Cook on both sides in a non-stick frying pan on medium heat until golden brown. Sprinkle cinnamon on top. Add small pat of margarine if you like.

Making a Bean-Sprouter

You will enjoy growing your own nutritious sprouts. It's easy and takes minimal effort. Just follow the steps presented below.

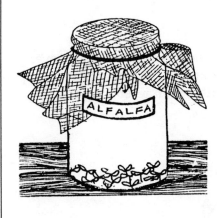

1. Put a handful of beans in the bottom of a clean quart-sized jar. (For alfalfa, put in only enough seeds to cover the bottom of the jar.)
2. Add enough water to cover the beans.
3. With a rubberband, fasten a piece of cheese-cloth over the mouth of the jar.
4. Soak overnight (for small seeds, such as alfalfa, soak for 3-4 hours).
5. Pour out the water. This water is excellent for soups and stews or for watering plants.
6. Put the jar in a cabinet or other dark place for 2-3 days. Rinse twice a day.
7. Place the jar on its side on a windowsill. Rinse twice a day until the leaves turn green.
8. Beans and legumes are best eaten when the sprouts are 1/4-1/2 inch long.
9. To prevent souring, rinse beans 3-4 times day.
10. Add low-calorie bean sprouts to soups, sandwiches, and salads.

One cup of alfalfa sprouts has 41 calories; one cup of mung, 37; one cup of soybeans, 48; one cup of lentils, 104.

Potato Cheesy Soup

1 medium potato, peeled and diced
1/3 cup water
2/3 cup skim milk
2 tablespoons fresh cheddar cheese, grated

Serves: 1

Slowly boil potato in water. When soft, drain. Mash in skim milk and cheddar cheese. Serve hot.

Stir-Fried Beef

1 tablespoon vegetable oil
1/2 cup lean sirloin, sliced thin
1/2 cup carrots, sliced diagonally
1/4 cup snow peas
1/4 cup water chestnuts

Serves: 1

Heat the oil in a non-stick frying pan or wok. Add beef and quickly brown. Remove. Add vegetables to pan and stir. Let cook for one minute. Return the browned meat to the pan and mix thoroughly with the vegetables. Let cook another minute, stirring occasionally. Serve hot over brown rice or any other cooked grain.

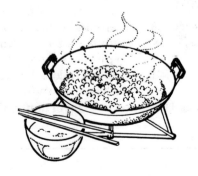

Snacks for Better Milk

Better Butter

1/2 teaspoon salt
2 tablespoons water
1 cup safflower, soy, or corn oil
1 cup softened butter (not melted)
2 tablespoons powdered skim milk
1/4 teaspoon lecithin

Yield: Approximately 3 cups

Mix salt and walter in a blender until salt is dissolved. Add all other ingredients and blend until smooth. Pour into containers and store in the refrigerator. (Recipe may be halved.) This is wonderful on whole-wheat or rye toast. (38 calories per teaspoon)

Fresh Vegetable Dip
---

1 teaspoon dill weed or seeds
1/3 cup cottage cheese
Low-fat milk
1/2 teaspoon spice(s) of choice
(eg. garlic powder, onion powder)

Yield: Approximately 1 cup

Whirl dill in the blender with cottage cheese and enough milk to make a creamy consistency. Add spices. Use this low-calorie (under 100!) dip for raw carrot and celery sticks, broccoli and cauliflower flowerets, green and red pepper rings, and mushrooms.

Nutritious and Fun Snacks

Fruity Milkshake

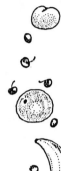

1 cup low-fat milk
2 ice cubes
any 2 of the following fruits:
1/2 banana
10 strawberries
1/4 cup blueberries
1/2 orange
1/2 nectarine

Yield: 1 large shake

Pour milk into a blender. Add ice cubes and fruit. Blend for 1-2 minutes. This quick, sweet, and satisfying snack is approximately 100-120 calories, but it is high in calcium, vitamins, and minerals.

Snack Suggestions

Satisfying, nutritious, and low in calories, the following snacks are excellent choices for the postpartum woman:

- 1 large, hard-boiled egg (82 calories)
- 1/2 cup frozen vanilla yogurt (120 calories)
- 6 ounces V-8 juice (35 calories)
- 1 ounce Swiss cheese (100 calories)
- 1/2 cantaloupe (40 calories)
- 1/3 cup cottage cheese (80 calories)
- 1 medium apple (82 calories)
- 1 small nectarine (40 calories)
- 1 small orange (60 calories)
- 4 ounces plain yogurt (100 calories)

Quick-Energy Snack

1/2 cup raisins
1/2 cup chopped dates
10 figs, dried
1/4 cup sunflower seeds
1/4 cup walnuts
1/4 cup unsweetened coconut
1/4 cup sesame seeds
(Substitute or add any other dried fruit, nuts, and seeds)

Yield: 24 small pieces
(73 calories each)

In a food processor, chop all the fruit, which will turn into a large, sticky ball. Remove the ball of fruit and set aside. Chop the remaining ingredients in the food processor, adding small pieces from the chopped fruit ball. When all the fruit has been added, put 2 tablespoons at a time into a plastic bag. Shape into a patty. Refrigerate. Break off pieces to eat as desired. Two or three pieces will give you a lift.

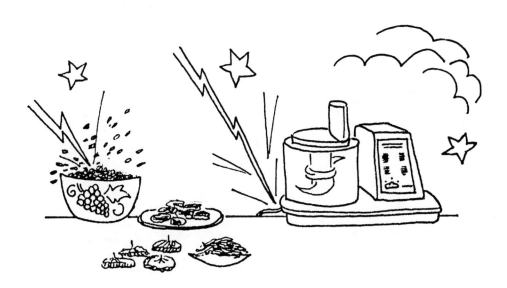

CHAPTER SIX

A Primer for the Nursing Mother

Your female body has the perfect equipment to enable your baby to grow and prosper. However, you have to "learn" how to nurse your baby so that you become a compatible team. For most "teams" it takes about two weeks to reach this state. Many women expect to be able to breastfeed their babies without any prior preparation or information. Some do very well on sheer luck, but many others are disappointed when breastfeeding doesn't match their previously imagined mental images. It takes some time and effort to adjust to the daily use of your breasts for feeding your baby.

Many women don't realize just how much time is spent feeding a newborn (breastfeeding and bottle-feeding) during the early weeks of a baby's life. Nursing a baby allows you a scheduled relaxation time that can help your postpartum body to heal. Mentally, however, you may want to be doing something other than sitting and resting while your baby feeds. Nursing then becomes a form of discipline. It forces you to calm down, relax, and take time for your baby and yourself as a team.

BASIC INFORMATION ON SUCCESSFUL BREASTFEEDING

Babies are born with the *rooting reflex*. If you touch them on the right cheek, they will turn to the right. Usually, if you touch your baby on the cheek nearest your waiting breast, the rooting reflex will cause the baby to look for the nipple. Squeezing on your breast a bit will cause the nipple to protrude making it more easily available to your infant. The baby should take both the nipple and a good section of the areola (brown part) into his mouth. During the first few days after birth, the baby should be fed on demand or at least every two to three hours (with a longer stretch at night) for a minimum of five to ten minutes on each breast. The more often you nurse your baby, the more quickly your nipples will toughen up. Frequent nursing will also insure that your milk supply will be plentiful for your baby.

While you're feeding your baby, you should hold him or her securely. Newborns like to be snugly wrapped in their receiving blankets. The firmness of the blankets, the warmth from your body, and the sound of your heartbeat remind the baby of his early life inside your uterus. It is extremely important to keep your baby physically close for some part of each day during the first few weeks. This is especially true for infants born via Cesarean section. Research has shown that this contact can be very healing and beneficial for infants who have not experienced a vaginal birth. This closeness will give your baby a sense of security and it will give you time to get to know your new child.

CORRECT BABY POSITIONING TO ELIMINATE SORE NIPPLES

When learning to breastfeed your baby, you may experience very sore nipples if your baby is positioned incorrectly. Try to follow these simple rules for correct baby position- ing to insure that breastfeeding is a rewarding experience.

1.   Wash your hands.
2.   Hold your baby in the crook of your arm, with your hand on your baby's buttocks or upper thigh.
3.   Hold your breast by placing four fingers beneath it and your thumb on top, making sure that your hand is not on the areola. *Do not* tilt the nipple up because this will incorrectly position your nipple in the baby's mouth and cause sore nipples.
4.   Bring your baby to the breast, *not your breast to the baby*. Point the nipple down and lightly tickle the baby's lower lip. Your baby should open his mouth as if he is yawn- ing.
5.   Pull your baby close and put him on the breast, not just on the nipple. Your baby's *hips, stomach, and head should face your body at the level of the breast*. You may need pillows and the arm of your rocking chair for support and comfort.
6.   If you had a Cesarean section, place pillows beneath your abdomen. Have your baby on his side facing you. Roll toward the baby, placing the entire breast in baby's mouth. You can use a bath pan at the foot of the bed to support your legs and prevent slipping down in bed. Don't lean over to nurse in bed, for that will cause a sore back.

If you experience sore breasts or clogged ducts, you should adjust your baby's position at the breast so that the baby's chin or jaw exerts pressure on your least tender spots. To determine the sore spot, visualize your breast as if it were a clock (see Figure 6.1). Try not to nurse on the tender spot. If you breastfeed in certain different positions (see Nursing Positions, page 91), you can minimize further breast irritation.

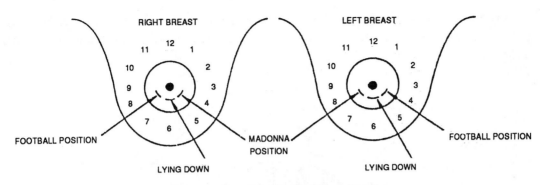

Figure 6.1 Position Rotation Chart

THE CURVED LINES INDICATE THE LOCATION OF SORE SPOTS ON THE NIPPLE OR AREOLA
CAUSED BY FREQUENTLY NURSING IN THE SAME POSITION.

Nursing Positions

Several different nursing positions are useful in preventing or eliminating breast soreness. The positions presented here are the most popular.

1. **The Front Hold** or **Madonna Position** (Figure 6.2). With pillows on your lap, sit up straight and cradle your baby in the crook of your arm with the baby's tummy against your chest.

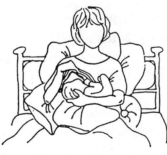

Figure 6.2 Front Hold or
Madonna Position

2. **The Football Hold** (Figure 6.3). With pillows on your lap, sit up straight and tuck your baby under your arm so his legs are behind you.

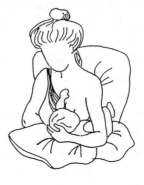

Figure 6.3 The Football Hold

3. Lying-Down Position (Figure 6.4). Lie on your side with pillows under your head, against your back, and between your legs. Have your baby lie on his side, facing you, with his mouth in line with your nipple.

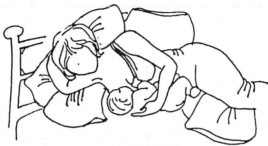

Figure 6.4 Lying-Down Position

PHYSICAL ASPECTS OF BREASTFEEDING

You may be surprised by the powerful sucking of your baby's tiny mouth. During the first few weeks of nursing, you may find that, as a result of this, your nipples are sore or tender. Continuation of nursing and proper positioning will help to eliminate the soreness (see Correct Baby Positioning on page 90 and Nursing Positions on page 91 for specific details).

Although you will be most aware of your breasts and nipples during the first days of the feeding process, you will soon begin to notice that there are other specific reactions occurring. Since your breasts were probably used in a sexual manner prior to your nursing time, you might find your body reacting with sexual-type feelings when you are breastfeeding.

Breastfeeding—like making love, conception, pregnancy, and delivery—is a sexual experience. Nipple erection usually occurs with sexual arousal as well as during breastfeeding. A hormone called *oxytocin* plays a role in both breastfeeding and in orgasm. It is not surprising then that some women report experiencing varying degrees of sexual stimulation such as clitoral sensations, increased sexual desire, and even orgasm during breastfeeding. Other nursing mothers report no sexual stimulation at all.

Many of my students have reported experiencing very pleasurable sensations while feeding their babies. They often, very quietly and shyly, ask if this is a normal reaction. This answer is a resounding "yes." The sexual parts of the female body usually react in unison when one section is stimulated.

Sometimes a student will ask, "What should I do about it?" "Enjoy these feelings!" is my answer. The mixture of sexual feelings and the warmth and smell of your baby adds immeasurable enjoyment to the nursing experience. Do not waste mental energy feeling guilty about the natural physical reactions of your female body.

SEX AND BREASTFEEDING

Although some women experience increased sexual desire during lactation, many others have a decreased desire for lovemaking. The skin-to-skin contact with the baby all day often decreases a woman's desire for more sexual contact. The lower estrogen levels in postpartum women can also decrease sex drive.

There is good evidence that nursing, when supported by your mate, improves bonding between mother, father, and baby. It enhances the relationship of the couple in the broader aspects of sexuality. Many women find a nurturing, supportive man to be a "turn on."

When resuming sexual activity, the following comments and suggestions may be of help:

- Nursing your baby before making love can help prevent the leaking of milk that often occurs during orgasm or nipple stimulation.
- Wearing a nursing bra and a nightgown might be helpful to prevent leaking.
- Fatigue may interfere with your sexual desire . . . just too tired to make love.
- You will probably experience some decrease in vaginal lubrication during lactation because of low estrogen levels. Using a water-soluble vaginal lubricant may increase your comfort and that of your mate.
- You may not experience an orgasm the first few times you have sexual relations after the baby is born. Relax. It will happen (sometimes even better than before you became pregnant).
- Finding time for lovemaking may also be a challenge. Making love early in the morning or when the baby is napping may work. You should plan intimate times together, as well as rest times, in order to increase your energy levels for each other.
- Many women are easily distracted during sex because their minds are on their babies. This does not indicate lack of interest or love for your partner but rather more interest in your new role as mother. As you become more relaxed as a mother, you'll find your distractions fewer and your interest in sex renewed.
- New dads may have difficulty in resuming lovemaking as before. Overwork and night feedings may cause overexhaustion in fathers, too! Talk out your feelings with your partner so that adjustments can be made.
- The support of your mate is essential to your success in breastfeeding. Fathers need physical loving so they don't resent the mother's attentiveness to the baby. Loving activities such as cuddling, kissing, and massages can help a new father feel important; it should help him be more supportive. There *is* sex after you have had a baby! And it will get better as the baby gets older.
- Breastfeeding is *not* a reliable contraceptive. Please refer to the discussion of contraception in Chapter Seven.

YOUR MENTAL ATTITUDE ABOUT BREASTFEEDING

The approach of taking each moment, each day, each week as it comes is extremely important when you're breastfeeding. Many women want to nurse their babies for a long time. However, with many women returning to work shortly after giving birth, many babies are only partially breastfed while they receive supplemental formula or the mother's previously pumped milk. Some women find that they are not able to totally nurse their babies for any of a variety of personal reasons. These women's guilty thoughts need to be explored and modified. Some of my students have faced these circumstances and have put themselves through extensive mental strain and tension while trying to accept the situation.

I can vividly recall a phone call from an agitated student. She had been nursing her son, but he had not been gaining weight and was often quite fussy during the day. After consulting with her pediatrician, she was able to nurse as often as possible and supplement her baby's diet with formula. Her adjustment to the physical aspect of this situation was quick and easy, but her mental feelings of guilt and inadequacy took a longer time to work through. After long discussions with her pediatrician, her husband, and me, she was finally able to accept that she was playing her mother role very well. She had previously believed that "good" mothering could only be accomplished by total breastfeeding. Once she was able to let go of her old beliefs and attitudes she was able to thrive as a loving mother. Learning to have faith in your own innate abilities and instincts, as well as having a flexible attitude or mindset can make your life so much easier and more enjoyable.

YOUR PARTNER'S ATTITUDE ABOUT BREASTFEEDING

Many new mothers find that their relationship with their partners changes drastically after the baby comes. Often, your mate can feel left out during the first few weeks postpartum because you may be exclusively taking care of your baby. The only way for a new father to learn his fathering role is if you give him a chance. By sharing some of the baby responsibilities, your mate can get to know his son or daughter while giving you some needed time off. After the baby finishes nursing on one side, encourage your mate to burp, change, and play with him until it's time to nurse again. Encouraging your husband to get involved with both you and the new baby will give you all a sense of the new family that has been created. Fostering a sense of closeness, warmth, and family from the very beginning will prevent your partner from feeling left out.

Both mothers and fathers have to make many mental and emotional adjustments to breastfeeding. Many new fathers have never seen a baby breastfeeding until their own baby is born. Seeing a baby feeding from an area of the female body that had been the husband's exclusive territory can cause some difficult and often unexpressed reactions.

Some fathers find that they are actually jealous of the baby's complete use of the breast. Some are upset because breasts may be less sensitive to stimulation during the nursing period or concerned because breasts may be tender the first few weeks. This doesn't mean breasts should be off limits. Frankly discuss this situation with your mate. Once he discusses his feelings openly, you can both come to conclusions that you find acceptable and agreeable. Many new fathers find feeding the baby a bottle of previously pumped breast milk or formula gives them a sense of usefulness while curbing some of their negative feelings. You may find other creative solutions. Openly facing and discussing negative feelings often eliminates more complicated problems later on. Remember, when you encourage your mate to spend time with the baby, you allow him to become a father and learn the skills involved in the process. He will also develop his own personal style with the baby that will be different from yours.

Many of my students find it very enjoyable is to have a "loving." My husband and I made up the term when my first son was born. A loving is a family hug. All the members of the family (even the dog) share the warmth and loving feelings of everyone else. You can have a loving simply by nursing your baby in bed while your husband hugs you. If you have another child, you can invite him or her to join. The physical contact and positive feelings of family lovings in my family are wonderful to experience. We continue to have them, even now that my sons are grown, because they are symbols of our family and the love that we feel for each other. Take a few minutes each day to enjoy and experience these pleasurable feelings with your new family.

HELPFUL EQUIPMENT FOR BREASTFEEDING

Although nursing is a natural experience, it is a learned skill. Here are several items that you may find useful:

- **A Rocking chair.** Since the baby was used to being rocked inside your uterus during pregnancy, the movement of a rocking chair during breastfeeding can be very relaxing. When choosing a chair, make sure the back is high enough to support your head and the arms are at the proper height for maximum comfort while you're holding your baby. Foam pads on the seat and the back of the chair should increase your comfort. Putting your feet up on an ottoman while nursing will help your circulation and will contribute to a relaxed feeling while breastfeeding. A calm and relaxed mother has a very positive influence on her baby and her breastfeeding experience.
- **Breast pumps.** These can be used to empty your breasts when they are too full or engorged with milk. They can also be used to pump out milk that will be used when you are away from your baby. Extra milk can be refrigerated for up to two weeks or deep frozen from six months to two years. Today, there are many styles of breast pumps available, some with detachable bottles for easy and quick milk collections. Breast pumps are available through the *Be Healthy* catalog (page 307).

• **Breast shields.**   These ventilated, feather-light plastic shields are worn over your breasts inside your bra between feedings. They help inverted nipples come out and keep cracked nipples dry. They also keep your breasts from sticking to your bra or nursing pads.

• **Nursing pads.**   Many new mothers have leaking breasts. A variety of nursing pads are commercially available; however, clean, folded handkerchiefs are just as effective. Avoid those varieties with plastic liners; these will keep your nipples wet.

HELP FOR NURSING MOTHERS

Through the efforts of the La Leche League, counseling for all nursing mothers is just a phone call away. Check with your pediatrician or childbirth educator for the number of your local La Leche League leader. You would be wise to attend the monthly meetings of nursing mothers. Seeing other mothers nursing their babies and discussing common problems can be very reassuring. Generally, there are no fees for counseling or for meetings. The goal of the League is to educate women about the art of breastfeeding. The most complete, up-to-date book available on nursing is published by the La Leche League; it is entitled *The Womanly Art of Breastfeeding.* Check other listings under Breastfeeding in the Recommended Reading Section beginning on page 297.

CAUTIONS AND COMMENTS ON BREASTFEEDING

• Eat a balanced diet of four to six small meals daily. Add one extra serving of calcium-rich foods such as milk, tofu, and sesame seeds.
• Keep a glass of water, herbal tea, milk, or juice near you to drink as you nurse.
• To induce calmness and better milk production, try adding one tablespoon of Brewer's yeast to one eight-ounce glass of tomato juice. Drink this mixture three times a day.
• Carry a receiving blanket to put over your shoulder and partly over the baby for nursing discreetly.
• *Do not pull the baby off the breast.* Press the breast gently away from the corner of the baby's mouth with your fingers until the suction is broken.
• Do not be mentally agitated by comments such as: "When are you going to get your baby on a bottle?" or "How long do you intend to keep feeding your child *that* way?" Always answer in a positive way—"As long as both of us enjoy it," or "My child is thriving and happy with this system," or "My baby sleeps well."
• Do enjoy the supreme usefulness of your feminine body.
• Think about your own self-image and how it is enhanced by the knowledge that your body can provide nourishment for your child.

- Do not feel depressed if you need to supplement your breastfeeding with formula. Some babies require this. It is not an indication that you are a "poor" mother. You are doing the best job that you can.
- Do not take any drugs when you are nursing without checking with your caregiver to see if the drug is on the approved list.
- Do not drink alcohol excessively, for your baby will receive a large dose of alcohol via your milk.
- Do not exercise before nursing. Exercise can cause the milk to become highly acidic; baby will not like the taste.
- Be aware that all things that you eat and drink become part of your milk, so try to limit heavily spiced or gassy foods.
- Do ten to fifteen rounds of Abdominal Breaths (page 17) when you are having difficulty settling down to feed your child.
- Do not have preconceived notions about how long you will nurse before adding solid food to your baby's diet.
- Take things as they come and you will not be disappointed.
- Have faith in yourself and your abilities to nourish and nurture your child.

As you can see, there is a very strong relationship between successful nursing and being able to relax at will. Sometimes you will have to nurse your baby when you have a mile-long list of things to do! Yet you will have to drop everything and satisfy your child. One of the most beneficial advantages of nursing your baby is forced relaxation time each day while the baby is feeding. The closeness, warmth, and pleasurable feelings that you will experience while breastfeeding are an extra special bonus of motherhood. Enjoy!

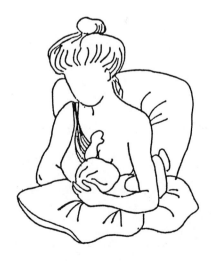

CHAPTER SEVEN

Reawakening Your Sexual Self

"Somewhere between the hospital and my house, I lost my sexual drive!" "I'm afraid my sex drive will never come back." "I'm just not in the mood very often." "I am thinking about my baby while we're trying to make love." "I am so tired by ten o'clock, I'd rather go to sleep." "My stitches still hurt, and lovemaking just makes it worse." These are common responses to the question, "How is your sex life?" For weeks and sometimes months after the baby arrives, one other very popular answer to this question is, "What sex life?"

You may be laughing or sighing with relief as you read these comments because you may relate to them. You may feel that there is just not enough energy right now for two complete roles—wife and mother. Learning to blend these two roles, being a wife one minute and a mother the next, takes some practice. Initially, many women have difficulty re-establishing their sex lives for the reasons just mentioned. Some sense a conflict between being a loving and devoted mommy and being a sexy woman, while others gain total satisfaction just from taking care of the baby. Some mothers don't realize that circumstances and reactions change daily. Have patience and faith that things will improve.

POSTPARTUM PHYSIOLOGICAL CHANGES

You should be aware of the natural physiological changes within your body immediately following the birth of your child. The following can help ease your mind concerning your sexual response:
- Until your period returns, you may experience decreased sexual desire due to low estrogen levels in your body.

- You may experience weak, sexually unresponsive pelvic floor muscles with lowered vaginal lubrication when lovemaking. This can occur any time from one month to two years postpartum. Using vaginal jelly or cream can eliminate this problem.
- If you are nursing your baby, you may have to wear a nursing bra (which is not very sexy) while making love.
- Your body, not listening to your mind at all, might let your milk down, thereby giving you and your mate a milk bath!
- You may subconsciously believe that your breasts should only be used by your baby and not for a sexual response.
- You may actually believe that mothers cannot be sexy.
- You may have much difficulty concentrating and then letting go and reaching orgasm, because mentally you may be listening for your baby.
- Often you may be too tired to have any sexual response because of nighttime feedings.
- Your healing process in the vaginal or abdominal areas may be slow, causing pain or burning sensations rather than the usual pleasurable responses associated with sex.
- You may not want to be touched after being close to your baby all during the day.
- You may have difficulty discussing your feelings honestly and openly with your mate.

For first-time mothers these startling physical and emotional reactions, coupled with the responsibility of a new baby, can cause very discouraging thoughts and feelings. Once you realize that your responses are normal and acceptable, you will be able to do something about the situation. Some women adjust and heal very quickly, thus resuming their sex lives relatively quickly. The idea of abstaining from sex until the six-week check-up is old-fashioned; many caregivers now advise women to resume sexual relations as soon as they feel comfortable and ready.

ADVICE FROM AN EXPERT

According to Pamela Shrock, PhD, childbirth educator and sexual counselor, many postpartum women feel overwhelmed by the enormous responsibility of taking care of a newborn. Such a woman needs to recognize that the first few months of fatigue, insecurity in this new role as mother, and lack of time for herself, let alone for her relationship with her husband, will not last forever.

There are times when a woman may feel that the amount of love she has to give is a fixed quantity. While giving so much of herself to her baby, she cannot imagine having any love left to give to her husband. Oftentimes, he may sense this and feel left out; he may blame her for excluding him. So the baby may become an object of rivalry and conflict, separating the parents rather than strengthening their bond.

Being able to express these feelings and to discuss the hurt, the anger, the feelings of being left out, of being overwhelmed, or of just being scared or afraid helps the couple face these minor irritations before they grow into major conflicts. Timely discussions will often prevent these upsets from affecting the couple's ability to share love and intimacy.

A woman may be resentful and blame her husband for her pregnancy. The pregnancy may have interfered with career plans or caused financial strain. Her anger and resentment may cause her to retaliate by being sexually distant, not having intercourse, and even withholding her own sexual arousal.

A woman may become confused when she experiences natural and normal sexual arousal while breastfeeding her baby. She may perceive this as wrong, sinful, or bad. If she is not made aware that nipple stimulation often leads to reflex arousal, her anxiety may lead to her blocking her sexual feelings.

Parents, fearful of another pregnancy, may avoid intercourse. Use of birth control may not be feasible during those early weeks, so couples need to develop different forms of expressing their sexuality. They need to become intimate or give pleasure to one another in ways other than intercourse.

Discussing these feelings with one another, having a sense of humor, being there for one another, supporting and cheering one another on, and showing loving affection helps the couple maintain sexual health and a solid relationship.

DAILY CLEANLINESS

One very simple way to increase your femininity and desirability is to shower or bathe at least once a day. If you are lucky, on some days you may find a few spare moments for a second shower. Being clean is a very effective way to increase your own desirability. The warm water will not only cleanse you physically, but it is a good technique for emotional cleansing, too. A shower or bath may be the only time during the day when you have a few minutes to yourself. It is at this time that you can dwell on your femininity and let it grow. These private moments can and should be very precious to a new mother who is on call twenty-four hours a day. By cleansing your body and hair, you will feel restored and refreshed.

It is important after the first two weeks postpartum to get dressed each day. You may still be wearing some maternity clothes at this time, but don't despair. Your prepregnancy figure will come back in time. Getting yourself washed and dressed can contribute to your own self-esteem and attractiveness. The mental connection between feeling desirable and sexual functioning is a well-known fact.

EXERCISES FOR REAWAKENING YOUR SEXUAL SELF

After developing a routine of daily cleanliness, it is important to resume your practice of several Positive Parenting Fitness exercises that can contribute to healing, toning, and stimulating your sexual organs, your hormonal system, and your entire body, especially your sexual self. The most effective exercises for gently reawakening your sexual area are presented in the following list:

- The Abdominal Lift (page 139)
- The Bridge (page 132)
- The Fish (page 149)
- The Shoulderstand (page 144)
- The Sitting Spinal Twist (page 140)

In addition, the following exercises are specifically designed to help reawaken your sexuality after your baby is born. Gently exercising the genital area will speed the healing process while strengthening the perineal muscles. This will bring back tone and responsiveness. Your partner will surely appreciate your effort!

The Squeeze with Baby

Benefits

- Tightens and helps heal the pelvic floor (bulbospongiosus, transverse perinei superficialis, profundus, and ischiocavernosus) while restoring muscle function
- Shapes the buttocks
- Prevents constipation and hemorroids
- Eliminates the incompetent bladder symptoms that result from relaxation of the pelvic floor muscles
- Increases sexual pleasure

Directions

1. Lie on your back with your feet crossed at the ankle. Your baby should be on your chest or held above your chest.
2. Flatten your lower back into the mat by tilting your pelvis.
3. Inhale fully. Exhale and contract your entire pelvic floor—the urinary tract, the vaginal muscles, and the anal muscles. (Figure 7.1)
4. Hold for ten seconds.
5. Inhale and repeat 5-10 times.

Cautions and Comments

- This exercise should be practiced immediately after your baby's birth, but repetitions should be limited to five times every waking hour. In time, repetitions should be increased.
- Practice just as you drift off to sleep at night.
- Practice this exercise while in a Shoulderstand (page 144).

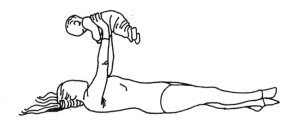

Figure 7.1 The Squeeze (with baby)

The Elevator

Benefits

- Exercises and strengthens all the inner muscles of the pelvic floor
- Helps keep the genital area invigorated and responsive

Directions

1. In any comfortable position with your legs separated, become aware of your vaginal muscles.
2. Imaging that your pelvic floor muscles are an elevator that is slowly moving from the first to the sixth floor as you slowly pull your muscles up toward your spine. You may feel a slight tightening sensation in the lowest part of your tummy.
3. Really concentrate and feel the muscles on the first floor, second, etc. Hold the elevator at the sixth floor for 5-10 seconds and then slowly allow this elevator to descend.
4. Control the descent to the first floor and then lower it to the basement by pushing downwards.
5. Repeat the trip 2-3 times then relax by taking several Abdominal Breaths (page 17).

Cautions and Comments

- As your muscle tone increases, it will become much easier for you to hold the elevator on the top floor.
- This exercise is often called a "vaginal handshake" or "clasp" and can easily be practiced while making love. Both partners benefit from practice at that time, for the upper third of the vagina has different sensations from the lower. Practice and find out . . . .

Kegels (Pelvic Floor Exercises)

Benefits

- Promotes speedy healing of the episiotomy incision
- Prevents urine leakage
- Helps restore muscle tone to the vaginal muscles
- Helps reduce swelling
- Helps reawaken sexual drive
- Stimulates pelvic activity; strengthening and toning the pelvic floor will lead to increased sexual pleasure
- Strengthens bladder sphincters to urethra
- Strengthens pelvic floor (bulbospongiosus, transverse perinei superficialis and profundus, sphincter urethrae, and ischiocavernosus)

Directions

1. When you urinate, after passing half of the urine, stop the flow.
2. Close your eyes and feel the contracted pelvic floor muscles.
3. Urinate a bit more and then contract again.
4. Repeat this contraction of the pelvic floor 4-5 times every time you urinate.
5. Once you know how to contract these muscles, perform this exercise several times a day when you are not urinating. Hold each contraction for 2 seconds until you work up to 50 Kegels a day (5 sets of 10). This sounds like a lot of work, but it really takes very little time.

Cautions and Comments

- These exercises should be started right after the baby is born; they should be done throughout the hospital stay and continued when you return home.
- Learn to rely on your abdominal muscles as a supportive splint by tightening them when you are moving or standing.
- Practice Kegels while feeding the baby, when watching TV, while talking on the phone, etc.

Tapus or Heating Breath

Benefits

- Develops your power of concentration
- Strengthens the vaginal and abdominal areas
- With some practice, this exercise can help awaken and revitalize your genital area

Directions

1. Assume a comfortable position; close your eyes, inhale slowly through your nose.
2. As you exhale, imagine a small opening between your vagina and your anus, through which you feel the air being exhaled. Push down and forward with your vaginal muscles as you exhale. Get every bit of air out.
3. Imagine that the air you are exhaling is stimulating, toning, and energizing your sexual self.
4. Repeat 5-15 times.

Cautions and Comments

- This is a very dynamic breathing exercise that, if practiced faithfully, can stimulate and wake up your genital region.
- Practice this while feeding your baby.
- Sometimes this exercise will result in a feeling of heat in the sexual region, thus the name Heating Breath.

MASSAGE FOR SENSUAL AROUSAL

A heightened sense of sexual arousal can be experienced if lovemaking is preceded by a pleasant body massage. Sometimes, because of a shortage of time or a crying baby, a massage can be a substitute for making love. The following massage need not take very long but is well worth the effort for a more positive sexual experience.

Often with a baby's erratic schedule, there is little time for elaborate massage preparations. Keep some oil near your bed. Use vegetable oil, preferably almond or sesame because it is readily absorbed into the skin. (Baby oil clogs pores.) Begin the massage by deciding who is going to give and who is going to receive. If you find your sexual desire flagging, it might be a good idea to receive.

Simple Massage Rules

- When using different massage strokes, glide from one stroke to another as smoothly as you can.

- Try to mold your hands to your partner's body.

- Vary the speed and pressure of your strokes but do so smoothly.

- The person who is receiving should be passive and should not try to help during the massage. The receiver should relax mentally and enjoy the sensations while keeping his or her eyes closed.

- Centering and tuning into the sensations is the receiver's job.

- If a massage is given for too long a period of time, in an irregular pattern, and/or without lubrication, the receiver can actually become more tense.

Preparing for the Massage

1. Choose a warm, quiet place.
2. Provide some relaxing music.
3. If time allows, light a candle to help create an intimate atmosphere.
4. Massages should not be given in bed because of the movement of the mattress; however, it is acceptable for short massages. Instead, perform massages on top of a blanket that has been placed on a carpeted floor. An oil sheet should be placed on top of the blanket to catch any spills.
5. Always use oil, talc, or corn starch for lubrication. Sesame, almond, safflower, and coconut oil are best absorbed by the skin. Scented oils are fun to use, too. (See Mail Order Products in the Appendix for ordering information.) The oil or talc will enable your hands to apply pressure while moving smoothly over the surface of the skin. Store the oil in a plastic container with a closeable top, and heat the bottle under warm water before use. Be aware that vegetable oils stain, so use old towels or sheets during massage.
6. The receiver of the massage should be nude. Keep a sheet or blanket handy in case of coolness during the massage or for modesty during an interruption.
7. Make sure your nails are short so as not to hurt your partner.

Popular Massage Strokes

When giving a massage it is best to vary the strokes as well as the pressure. Try the following popular massage strokes:

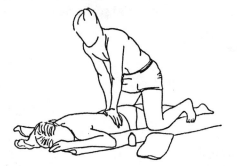

Palm-Pressure Stroke

With open hands, press down on the lower back and slowly move your hands out to the sides. Move up the spine with this stroke.

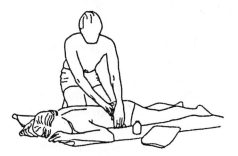

Hand-Over-Hand Stroke

Place one hand under your partner's side at the waist, and pull your hand back toward you with some pressure. Follow with a second hand as you move up the side to the shoulder area. This should be done on both sides.

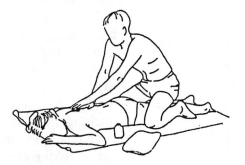

Double-Hand Stroke

Starting at the neck, move both hands (one on top of the other) down the back.

The Sensual Massage

Benefits

- Releases physical and emotional tension
- Heightens the bodily senses
- Encourages a sense of closeness between you and your partner
- It feels great!

Directions

1. If you are receiving the massage, lie on your abdomen on a soft blanket.
2. If you are giving the massage, begin by putting a small amount of oil in the palms of your hands. Rub your hands together until they are warm.
3. Begin to move your hands slowly up your partner's back starting at the base of the spine. Move your hands up the shoulders and then down the sides of the back. Repeat this "main stroke" 3-6 times (Figure 7.2). Add oil if needed.

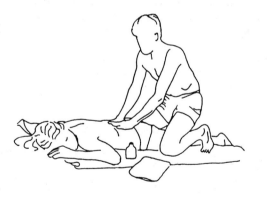

Figure 7.2   The "Main Stroke"

4. Next, place your oil-moistened hands at the bottom of the spine (near the buttocks) and massage in a circular motion with firm first pressure from 30 seconds to 2 minutes (Figure 7.3).

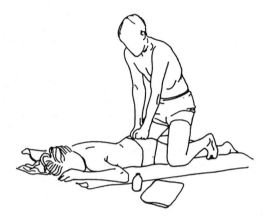

Figure 7.3   Using Fist Pressure

5. Using the same circular pressure, move your hands up from the buttocks and spend another minute or two massaging the lower back. Make sure your partner points out any sore or tender spots so you can spend more time (and less pressure) on these areas.
6. Now move your hands to either side of the spine but never on the spine itself, using either very firm or very light, teasing strokes.
7. Next, concentrate on your partner's upper back and neck by kneading the skin lightly between your fingers in a pinching motion (Figure 7.4). Since much tension is often felt in the neck and shoulder area, a full minute or two should be devoted to the massage here.

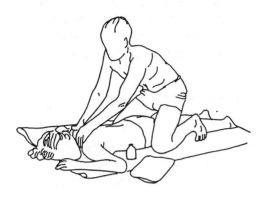

Figure 7.4 Massaging the Neck

10. Next, concentrate on the shoulders and neck. Find the tense spots and try to eliminate them by using consistent pressure.

11. The facial muscles, especially those around the mouth, are closely associated with the vaginal area. Therefore, a brief facial massage can be sexually stimulating. Beginning with the forehead, move your thumbs back and forth across this area(Figure 7.6) 2-3 times. Massage the cheeks. Massage the eye area carefully.

8. Now, have your partner turn over onto her back.

9. The upper back can be effectively massaged by sliding your hands under it, palms up, and pressing up with your fingers (Figure 7.5). Starting at the lower back, lift the chest up. Continue moving your fingers up the back lifting the chest as you go. Do this until the entire back is free from tension.

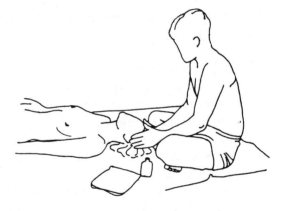

Figure 7.6 Massaging the Forehead

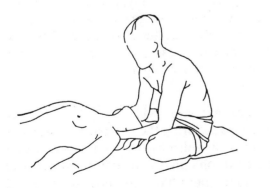

Figure 7.5 Relieving Upper-Back Tension

12. Move to the jaw and mouth area massaging gently.

13. Next, move to the neck and upper-chest area using a hand-over-hand movement.

14. Work the tensions from the chest area by moving your hands with some pressure several times over the chest and shoulders (Figure 7.7).

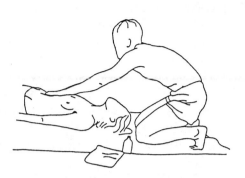

Figure 7.7   "Main Stroke" on the Chest

15.   Lightly tease the sexual area as part of the chest massage. This will heighten sexual arousal.
16.   Be creative. Go on to other areas of the body, using different techniques. Try the following:

• Brush the body with light finger strokes using all your fingers.
• Brush the body with one finger, tracing over the entire body.
• Pay more attention to those areas of your partner's body that are most easily aroused.
• Begin connecting the genitals with the rest of the body by lightly touching them and then going on to other parts of the body. This will gradually transfer the higher sexual arousal (usually associated only with the genitals) to the rest of your body.

• Using a bit of oil or vaginal jelly, massage the genital area very slowly and sensually (if it is fully healed).
• From this point, you should know what to do. . . . Have fun!

Cautions and Comments

• Invent your own massage techniques in order to increase your sexual response.
• If you are not completely healed, you can have sexual pleasure through methods other than intercourse. Manual stimulation can bring you and your mate to orgasm.
• The postpartum period of your life is a very good time to expand your sexual experiences.
• Discuss your feelings about massage, making love, tiredness, etc. openly and honestly with your partner. Don't assume that you will not be sexually responsive.
• Try making a date for mutual massage at a time you know (or at least hope) the baby will be asleep.
• Try to massage in a variety of rooms and during different times of the day.
• Have someone watch your baby so you can get away for a day, possibly to a motel, and try this massage technique.
• Have faith that this unresponsive time in your life will pass and your passionate self will return once again.

These simple massage techniques and physical exercises will help you gradually redevelop your sexual desires. The variety of responses during the postpartum period is vast, and it is difficult to say when your bodily responses will return to what you consider normal. These techniques should not be considered miraculous cures but positive and practical suggestions to help your postpartum adjustment. Working now to tone and reactivate your sexual nature can enrich and strengthen your marriage.

DEALING WITH DISCOMFORT

Many women find that the first few times they make love postpartum can be quite uncomfortable. It is advisable to use vaginal jelly the first time you resume relations even if you have never used vaginal jelly before. This extra lubrication is highly beneficial for reducing pressure on tender areas.

Several of my students have experimented in trying to find comfortable and satisfying positions. Many have said that a position where the woman is dominant is most comfortable for them. You may find as you resume a sexual relationship that you are more comfortable with shallow-penetration lovemaking positions. Many couples find *The Joy of Sex* by Alex Comfort, PhD, quite helpful for providing pleasurable new positions.

There are several books that can help you discover how other women and couples respond sexually during the postpartum period. *Making Love During Pregnancy* by Elizabeth Bing and Libby Coleman, *Sex After the Baby Comes* and *Women's Experience of Sex*, both by Sheila Kitzinger, will broaden your understanding of your sexual response or lack of it. See the Recommended Reading List (page 297) for additional titles.

You may find that time is scarce for sexual experimentation. Often a crying baby will change the mood that you and your partner have created. Within these limitations, the best advice is to do what you and your mate find most satisfying and pleasurable.

BIRTH CONTROL

If the information in this chapter is not useful to you because you are easily stimulated sexually, your reaction is also considered normal. Some postpartum women feel more feminine and responsive. It's important to realize, however, that your chances of becoming pregnant again are significantly greater if your sexual drive is high. Since so much of this chapter concerns sexual stimulation, this is an appropriate time to discuss birth control. Please, read this section carefully and remember:

- You *can* conceive a baby when you are breastfeeding.
- You must be refitted with a new diaphragm or cervical cap after the baby's birth even if you have had a Cesarean section.
- You cannot use birth control pills when you are breastfeeding.

It is difficult to know just when you will ovulate again once you have had your baby. This is why you should use a specific method of birth control as soon as you resume sexual relations. Usually your caregiver will discuss this decision with you at the time of your six-week check-up. However, you and your partner may make love sooner. If you do, your partner can use a condom and you can use vaginal jelly or foam.

A variety of birth control methods are available. You and your spouse should discuss and agree on the best method(s) for you.

Cervical cap. A small barrier device, the cervical cap is filled with spermicidal jelly or cream and placed over the cervix. If used correctly, this method is 97 percent effective.

Condom. A condom is a rubber device shaped to fit over the erect penis iń order to prevent sperm from entering the vagina. When used correctly, this method of birth control is 97 percent effective; it also provides protection from sexually transmitted diseases.

Contraceptive implant. A set of capsules that prevents ovulation is inserted under the skin of a woman's arm and is effective for up to five years. This method is reported to be almost 100 percent effective.

Diaphragm. A diaphragm is a rubber cup that is placed in the vagina to form a barrier between the uterus and the sperm. Spermicidal jelly or cream is used in combination with the diaphragm. If used correctly, this method is 97 percent effective.

Intrauterine device (IUD). This small plastic device is placed in the uterus by a doctor. This method is 95-99 percent effective; however, there is a risk of uterine perforation.

Natural family planning. Also known as "periodic abstinence," this method involves taking your temperature, checking vaginal secretions, and keeping an accurate record of menstrual periods in order to predict your fertile days. This method is reported to be 90-97 percent effective.

"The Pill." Daily doses of hormones in pill form prevent ovulation. Birth control pills are almost 100 percent effective. Note: "The pill" is not recommended for nursing mothers. There are, however, no studies that show any adverse side effects for infants whose mothers are using low-dose pills. Progesterone-only preparations show no definite changes in breast milk.

Spermicidal foam and condom. Spermicidal foam destroys sperm. When used in combination with a condom, this method is nearly 100 percent effective.

Spermicidal jellies, foams, and creams. Inserted directly into the vagina before intercourse, these spermicidal agents kill sperm. They are 89 percent effective; however, many women find them messy and inconvenient.

Sterilization. The ducts carrying the sperm or the egg are tied and cut (vasectomy or tubal ligation). Sterilization is almost 100 percent effective.

Vaginal sponge. A soft polyurethane sponge that is filled with spermicide, the vaginal sponge is placed in the vagina where it blocks and kills sperm. This method is 89 percent effective.

PART II

Positive Parenting Fitness Exercise Program

CHAPTER EIGHT
Program Overview and Guidelines

According to physical therapist Marilyn Freeman, who has worked extensively with postpartum women, the female body doesn't return to a "normal" prepregnancy state of the muscles, tendons, ligaments, and joints until at least nine months after the baby is born. If you are breastfeeding your hormonal levels will be elevated throughout the breastfeeding experience, and that may slow down your return to a more stable prepregnancy state. Each body is different and returns to its prepregnancy state at a different rate. When I was breastfeeding my sons, my body shed pounds and inches in record time. There are other facts about pregnancy and postpartum that you should be aware of before you start a "shape-up-after-baby" program.

According to Ann Cowlin, MA, director of the Dancing Thru Pregnancy and After program:

> *During pregnancy, your center of gravity gradually changes. Before pregnancy, your body weight is centered over your hips. As the baby grows, your center of gravity shifts so most of your weight is in front of your hips. This leads to changes in the arrangement of your spine. The natural S-curve deepens, and the vertebrae change position as the weight on the front of your belly increases. After childbirth, your goal is to gradually return the spine to its prepregnancy alignment.*

During pregnancy and right after delivery, your joints are more flexible and less secure. It may take three to six moths or more for these bodily changes to revert back to normal. The looseness of your joints and the exaggerated curve of your spine have to be taken into account when you consider your sleeping, sitting, standing, and moving postures. Therefore, postpartum is a *transitional phase* in which safeguards and rules have to be followed.

If you maintained good posture during your pregnancy, you may have fewer complaints after giving birth. If you exercised and did light weight training during your pregnancy, you should have a much easier time getting back into shape because you have maintained appropriate muscle tone. If you didn't exercise during your pregnancy, don't lose heart! The Positive Parenting Fitness program will ease you back into exercise safely and easily either by yourself or with your baby. Part III even includes stretches for fathers and babies so that new daddies don't feel left out!

POSTPARTUM POSTURE

Your posture is an obvious sign that tells the world how you feel. Good posture is a combination of appearance and function. It is largely controlled by a reflex or subconscious mechanism, but it is also affected by outside factors such as emotions, neglected or damaged muscles, and weight change. After pregnancy, your posture may be "stuck" in the pregnancy mode and you will have to re-educate your muscles.

Remember, your body had to adapt to a lot of changes during pregnancy. It had to accommodate increased body weight, accentuated spinal curves, and widened hips and pelvis. Your ligaments were also stretched to their maximum capacity.

Now that your baby is born, you will have to relearn how to stand and sit properly. Your body has amazing powers of rejuvenation, and those overstretched, overworked muscles will shorten and become more elastic *if you make a conscious effort to feel the muscles you are using when holding a proper posture.* Try to think about your posture as you stand, sit, and walk. When you feel you are displaying "good" posture, note the muscles that are working to hold it for you. By repeating both poor and proper postures, you will notice that the proper posture relieves tension (though it may feel unnatural at first). The more you repeat the proper posture, the more natural it will become.

When assessing your posture, look at yourself sideways in a full-length mirror. You might ask a friend to help you in your analysis.

Proper Postpartum Posture

As illustrated in Figure 8.1, good posture is characterized by the following:

•A head that is well-balanced; one that does not compress your neck. Pretend there is a string pulling your head toward the ceiling. The back of your neck should lengthen upward by elongating the posterior muscles.
•When your shoulders are relaxed and all tension is drained from your upper ex-tremities, there should be a straight line from your ear lobe to the tip of your shoulder.
•A spine that forms a gentle S-curve when standing. Your neck and lower back should curve gently toward your front while your upper back and rib cage should curve gently backward.

Tighten your buttocks and pull in your abdominal muscles as you tilt the top of your entire pelvis backward, moving your pubic bone slightly forward and upward.

Take a deep breath and expand your ribs upward and outward. Next, move your feet apart so that they align with your hips. Observe your posture in the mirror now. Make a mental note of how your body feels. This is how you should feel when your posture is good.

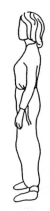

Figure 8.1   Proper Postpartum Posture

Poor Postpartum Posture

As illustrated in Figure 8.2 poor posture is characterized by the following:

• A chin that juts out so that your cervical spine is exaggerated forward (not in the natural S-curve).
• Rounded shoulders that increase the backward curve of your rib cage or thoracic spine.
• An arched lower back that can create backaches.
• Knees that are locked and hyperextended.
• An uneven distribution of body weight onto one leg, creating an unnatural shifting of your torso and a curving of your spine.

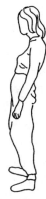

Figure 8.2   Poor Postpartum Posture

THE FOUR-STEP PROGRAM

It takes from three to six months for most women's bodies to adjust to the non-pregnant state and up to nine months to fully recover from pregnancy and childbirth. Because your body took a full nine months to stretch, grow, and produce a fine baby, a three to six month readjustment period is actually a short time. Keep in mind, however, that this process is *slow and gradual.* Your body is in a vulnerable state due to changing hormonal influences. As you are "on call" day and night with your baby, fatigue may also influence the bad habits of poor posture and body movements. Therefore, it is unreasonable to immediately throw your body into any extensive exercise such as running or high-impact aerobics.

The Positive Parenting Fitness program is a four-step program that will ease you back into shape gradually, the way nature intended. The four steps of this program should be followed in the order of their progression. They have been designed to ease your body back to its prepregnancy state.

Before detailing the actual exercises, each step of the program will be discussed. Guidelines will be set as well as Do's and Don'ts for each phase of the program.

Step #1 includes exercises for the first three to six weeks postpartum. These exercises are based primarily on stretching. The "Basic Eight" and the "Sun and Moon Salutes" naturally progress as Step #2 to ease you naturally into exercise with or without your baby. Stretching is your body's natural response to a cramped position in order to relieve tension in your muscles and joints. By urging your muscles to release their pull on your joints, stretching restores flexibility and encourages a free, revitalizing flow of blood to your muscles as they relax. Flexibility exercises realign your body's joints, improve your shape and posture, and enhance circulation and respiration, thereby improving nutrition to your body's cells and tissues. They also ensure that you relax properly and completely.

Once you feel that you have mastered these exercises from Step #2, then you can go on to Step #3, the "Complete Body Workout." This step promotes an increase in the efficiency of your cardiovascular system including your heart and lungs. This section includes directions for warm-up exercises, proper breathing techniques, low-impact aerobic exercises, as well as cool-down exercises at the end of your workout. Aerobic exercise strengthens your heart muscle so that an increased volume of blood is able to be pumped with fewer strokes. These exercises also burn calories.

Step #4, "Shaping Up and Strength Training for Motherhood Survival," employs the use of light weights and/or Dyna-Bands, which are effective for shaping up postpartum trouble spots while maintaining muscle tissue. The exercises found in Step #4 help in preventing postural and lower-back problems, loss of bone mass, and osteoporosis.

Each of the following four chapters is devoted to the four steps of the Positive Parenting Fitness program. Each chapter includes important information, guidelines, and Do's and Don'ts specifically geared for each particular step of the program. Much of this information is designed to prevent any injuries.

Please keep in mind that this program should start at the beginning with Step #1 before progressing on to the other steps. Do not begin in the middle of the program without the proper muscle preparation through stretching and breathing techniques. And *always* check with your health-care provider before starting *any* exercise program.

CHAPTER NINE

Step 1
Healing Exercises for
the First Six Weeks

During the first several weeks postpartum, you will experience enormous changes both physically and emotionally. With so many changes in your daily life, this is not the appropriate time to begin an extensive exercise program. However, there are exercises that include breathing and relaxation, which can be easily integrated into your new routine (once you have one!), exercises to enhance your physical and mental adjustment during the postpartum period. Within this book, the term "postpartum" refers to the time after the baby is born when the mother fully heals and regains her prepregnancy shape.

Your doctor or midwife may give you a series of exercises to practice in the hospital and at home. You can choose to follow their suggestions or integrate them with the following suggested exercises. Much disagreement exists regarding the value of exercise during the first three to six weeks postpartum. You will have to make your own decision about exercising. Some doctors believe that since the muscle tone in the abdominal area does not return before twenty-one to twenty-eight days after your baby arrives, exercising this area is not very beneficial. Another consideration during this time is your loss of sleep from taking care of a newborn twenty-four hours a day. You may feel you do not have the time to fit in an exercise period. Luckily, the most important exercises during this time can easily be practiced while you are feeding your baby. For example, by practicing Abdominal Breaths (page 17) while you feed your child, you can actually increase your physical and mental relaxation levels. If you are breastfeeding, this breath is a good way to encourage the let-down reflex and to enhance your nursing experience.

RECTI SEPARATION

Every new mother should check for separation of her recti (abdominal) muscles. Check on your condition, especially after a Cesarean section, three days postpartum. Lie on your back with your knees bent. Pull your abdominal muscles in, lift your head and shoulders, and stretch one arm as hard as you can toward your feet. Put the fingers of your other hand just below your navel. You will feel the bundles of muscles tighten (see Figure 9.1). How many fingers can you fit sideways into the separation? One or two fingers would be considered a slight separation. This slackness will tighten on its own. If three or more fingers can fit between the two bundles of muscle, you need to make a special effort to restore these abdominal muscles.

If you are a post-Cesarean mother, *do not* practice this exercise until your incision is relatively pain-free. You should not experience any pain while practicing.

Exercise for Recti Separation

Benefits

- Aids maximum tone in the recti muscles and discourages further separation
- Strengthens all of the abdominal muscle groups
- Limbers up the spine and makes it flexible
- Eliminates or minimizes postpartum backache
- Tones the central nervous system
- Tones and tightens the thighs
- Relieves neck strain

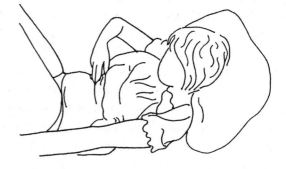

Figure 9.1   Checking for Recti Separation

Directions

1. Lying on your back, knees separated 12-16 inches apart, cross your hands over your abdominal area so that as you raise your head, you will be able to support the two recti muscles.
2. Breathe in deeply. Then exhale and raise your head forward to your chest, gently pushing the separated stomach muscles towards each other (see Figure 9.2).
3. You should practice this exercise to the point that you begin to feel a bulge.
4. Lower and repeat 3-5 times, twice a day.

Cautions and Comments

- The separation of your recti muscles is not a drastic situation. The hormones circulating in your body during pregnancy cause the central seam (linea alba) to soften and often separate. In addition, your stomach muscles are excessively stretched and strained during later pregnancy. A separation causes no pain, but you may suffer chronic backache throughout the pregnancy. You should always check on the status of your recti muscles.

• Protect your recti muscles by holding them throughout this exercise.

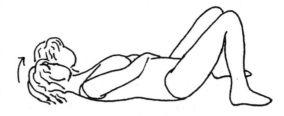

Figure 9.2 Exercise for Recti Separation

Healing Exercises After A Vaginal Birth

The following exercises can begin immediately after your baby is born. You can practice some of them while taking care of your baby.

Total Relaxation Exercise

Benefits

• Allows the pelvic organs to return to their normal positions as the weight of the body gently presses down on them
• Helps relieve episiotomy tenderness, hemorrhoids, and backaches
• Restores needed energy, which you can use when taking care of a newborn
• Helps relieve tension and brings about a sense of total relaxation

Directions

1. Lie flat on your stomach placing one pillow under your head and chest for support and a second pillow under your hips. Allow your breasts to fall freely between pillows (Figure 9.3). Face your head in either direction.
2. Let your legs fall comfortably into any position. Place your arms over your head or at your sides.
3. Rhythmically squeeze your buttocks 10-20 times. This helps relieve and heal post-delivery discomforts.
4. Take 1-2 Abdominal Breaths (page 17) and relax.
5. Remain in this position 15-30 minutes before slowly getting up.

Cautions and Comments

• Placing a pillow under your hips during this exercise reduces the arch in the small of your back, thereby minimizing strain in this area. You may even want to add a second pillow for more comfort.

- Use this position for your afternoon naps while your baby is sleeping.
- Do not lie in a tummy-down position without a pillow under your hips during the first week or two after delivery. It will place too much strain on ligaments and muscles of the lower back.
- Most women love this position because they have not been able to lie on their tummies for such a long time!
- Don't be tempted to prop yourself up on your elbows with your head raised in order to read. This position will put strain on your lower back.
- Cesarean-section mothers might find this position helpful and restful, too.

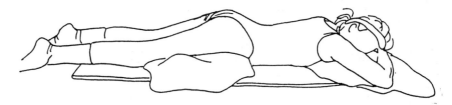

Figure 9.3   Total Relaxation Exercise

The Squeeze

Benefits

- Strengthens the anal sphincter muscles and part of the pelvic floor muscles; speeds healing of this area
- Aids in shrinking painful postpartum hemorrhoids

Directions

1. While standing under a warm shower, fold a washcloth until it is 4 x 1 inches. Wet the washcloth and wring it out.
2. Place the washcloth on the hemorrhoidal area and contract your anal muscles so that you are holding the washcloth with these muscles only. Hold the cloth for 5-10 seconds, then release.
3. Repeat 5-10 times.
4. After contracting and releasing the anal muscles, gently massage around the inflamed area with the washcloth.

Cautions and Comments

- The anal muscles, which are part of the pelvic floor muscles, tire easily, so you may choose to contract for very short intervals.
- Applying A and D ointment or vegetable oil to the hemorrhoidal area after your shower can be soothing.

Half Sit-Ups

Benefits

- Gently strengthens and firms the vertical abdominal muscles
- Strengthens the lower back, arms, and shoulders
- Firms buttocks
- Stretches cervical, thoracic, and lumbosacral erector spine muscles
- Strengthens deep anterior cervical paraspinals, sternocleidomastoids, and oblique abdominalis muscles; strengthens iliopsoas muscle group, gluteus maximus

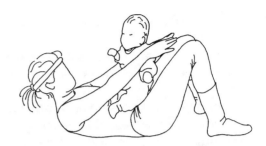

Figure 9.4   Half Sit-Up

Directions

1. Lie flat on your back with your knees bent and your feet on the floor about 8-10 inches apart. Rest your baby on your knees.
2. Raise both arms above your chest, on either side of your baby, raising your head and shoulders while you stretch up (Figure 9.4).
3. Hold this position, breathing normally, for 15-30 seconds or as long as is comfortable.
4. Slowly return to your starting position and take a breath.
5. Repeat 2-5 times, taking Abdominal Breaths (page 17) in between each Half Sit-Up.

Cautions and Comments

- Make sure you keep breathing while holding the Half Sit-Up. Some women find it more comfortable to pant or blow out through the mouth when holding this position.
- If you do not feel a definite pull on your abdominal muscles when stretching up, raise your chest and arms up a bit higher and closer to your knees.
- An effective variation of this exercise is to reach up over one knee, return to the starting position, breathe, then reach up over the other knee.
- As your baby gets older, you can practice this exercise with your baby resting on your stomach. Making faces at the baby as you hold the Half Sit-Up will encourage him to hold the position longer, thereby speeding up the return of a flat abdominal area.

Head-to-Knee Posture

Benefits

- Gently strengthens the abdominal muscles
- Relieves backache and sciatica while strengthening the lower part of the back
- Eliminates neck tension and stiffness
- Relieves flatulence and stomach gas
- Stimulates and improves digestion, promoting regular eliminations
- Stretches cervical, thoracic, lumbosacral erector spinae; glutei biceps femoris; and gastrocnemius of knee to chest
- Strengthens anterior cervical muscles, pectoral and biceps brachi, transverse and oblique abdominalis muscles

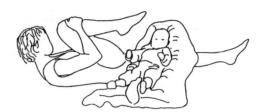

Figure 9.5   Head-to-Knee Posture

Directions

1. Lie flat on your back and take 1-2 Abdominal Breaths (page 17).
2. Slowly raise your left leg up into the air. Bend it at the knee and bring your knee down as close to your chest as possible.
3. Wrap your arms around your knee and pull it closer.
4. Now bring your forehead as close to your knee as you can and hold for 5-10 seconds (Figure 9.5).
5. Lower your head, release your arms, straighten your leg up into the air and gently but slowly lower it.
6. Take 1-2 deep breaths and repeat on the other side.
7. Repeat 2-3 times on each side.

Cautions and Comments

- This posture is invaluable when you have a gassy stomach. The knee-pressing movement will help move the gas down and out.
- Practice this posture with single legs until after the first two weeks postpartum. Then you can practice with both legs (one at a time).
- To hasten the contraction of your abdominal muscles, exhale when you are in the final position and hold 5-10 seconds before releasing.
- This is a very gentle but highly effective exercise.

Single Leg Lift with Baby

Benefits

- Gently strengthens weak abdominal muscles
- Massages and eliminates pain from the lower-back area
- Improves circulation, especially in the legs
- Helps tighten and firm the buttocks
- Stretches the thoraco-lumbar fascia, lumbo-sacral erector spinae, glutei biceps femoris, semimembranosus, semitendinosus, and gastrocnemius muscles
- Strengthens iliopsoas muscle groups, quadriceps (especially rectus femoris) adductors, oblique and transverse abdominalis muscles

Directions

1. Lying flat on your back, place the baby on your chest facing you. Take 1-2 Abdominal Breaths (page 17), and get ready to give your baby a ride.
2. Keeping your left leg straight on the floor, slowly begin to lift your right leg up into the air, taking 10-15 seconds to get it all the way up (Figure 9.6). As your leg is moving up, press the lower part of your back as close to the floor as possible.
3. Hold the leg upright for a count of 10 while breathing normally.
4. Take 15 seconds to return the leg to the mat.
5. Take 1-2 Abdominal Breaths (page 17) and repeat on the other side.
6. Practice 2-3 times on each side.

Cautions and Comments

- Moving the leg up and down quickly will not produce any benefits.
- Keep your leg straight as you raise and lower it.
- Focus on keeping your lower back on the mat.
- Do not hold your breath during this exercise; breathe normally.
- For an extra leg stretch, raise the leg with your foot flexed.

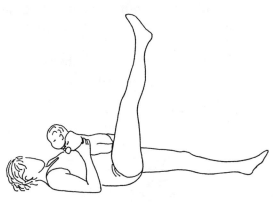

Figure 9.6 Single Leg Lift

Shoulder Circle and Shrugs

Benefits

- Eases tension and tiredness in the arms, shoulders, and upper back
- Stretches the upper thoracic postvertebrals, and the pectoralis major and triceps brachii muscles
- Tones and strengthens the biceps brachii, the middle deltoids, and the upper trapezius muscles

Directions

1. Extend your arms straight out to your sides.

2. From your shoulders, have each arm (at the same time) slowly make a large circle to the count of 10, then reverse the circle.

3. Now take an Abdominal Breath (page 17), lifting your shoulders as you inhale and lowering them as you exhale.

4. Repeat 10 times.

Cautions and Comments

- Tension is often stored in our neck and shoulders. This quick exercise will help relieve it.

Shoulder Stretch-Backs

Benefits

- Releases tension and tightness in the lower neck and upper and lower back, while strengthening these areas
- Develops and strengthens the pectoralis muscle group, which supports the breasts
- Strengthens middle trapezius, rhomboideus muscle groups; thoracic erector spinae muscles
- Stretches upper trapezius and spinalis muscles, the pectoralis major and minor muscle groups, and the subclavius muscles

Directions

1. Standing up straight, extend your arms to your sides, palms facing behind you.

2. Gently press your arms back 10 times as you exhale on every backward movement.

3. Next, clasp your hands behind you and lift them up while bending forward at the waist (Figure 9.7).

4. Repeat 3 times.

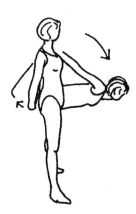

Figure 9.7   Shoulder Stretch-Backs

Cautions and Comments

• These shoulder exercises, if practiced often throughout the day, will help reduce or prevent shoulder tension and upper-back pain commonly caused by poor posture due to breastfeeding and general baby care.

Abdominal Breaths

See page 17 for complete directions.

Kegels

See page 104 for complete directions.

The Sitting Spinal Twist

See page 140 for complete directions.

After A Cesarean Delivery

A Cesarean delivery requires major surgery, therefore it takes considerably longer for your body to heal. Mentally you may tell yourself, "I'll never get back into shape; I'm so uncomfortable and ever so tired." If this is your attitude, please remember that realistically, a Cesarean-birth recovery is definitely more uncomfortable and prolonged than a vaginal-birth recovery. Although you may lag behind some other new mothers, you can start exercising now for comfort, healing, and muscle toning. Do remember you will experience more fatigue at first, so take it easy and keep a positive attitude.

Comfort Measures in the Hospital

In the hospital you might find your most comfortable position to be when you are propped up with pillows in a semi-reclining position. A pillow placed under your thighs will prevent you from sliding too far down in your bed. Adding another pillow across your incision will help avoid discomfort or pain when you breastfeed your baby; it is very important that you are in a comfortable and well-supported position.

Getting Out of Bed

Have your nurse lower your bed as close to the floor as possible. If you are lying flat, roll onto your side and prop yourself up on one elbow. Then use both arms to push yourself up into a sitting position. Edge toward the side of the bed, then, using your hands on your upper thighs, lift one leg at a time over the edge of your bed. Dangle your legs over the side for a few moments. As you stand up, support your Cesarean incision with one or both of your hands.

To get back into bed, make sure that the back of your bed is in an upright position. Using your pillows, brace your abdominal muscles while lifting your legs, one at a time, onto the bed.

Walking and Standing

When walking, you may lean over or stoop forward to protect your incision. But you will find that standing up straight, so the weight of your abdominal organs is off your incision, will be less painful. Gently supporting your wound with your hands will help ease the pain.

Learn to rely on the abdominal muscles as a "supportive splint" by voluntarily tightening them when changing positions or standing. This will encourage healing and help lessen post-surgical pain.

More Helpful Hints

Maureen Braun, RN, BN, and Positive Parenting Master Teacher, suggests the following information and exercises for post-Cesarean mothers in her Bodies and Babies classes.

Muscle Spasms

Initially after a Cesarean birth it will be hard to move. When you do, you may feel muscle spasms or painful abdominal contractions. (These muscles are tightening in order to protect themselves from further injury.) Relaxing those tightening muscles is very important for comfort.

Close your eyes and breathe gently, slowly, and deliberately into the painful area. To further concentrate on the muscle spasm, place your hands gently over the affected area and focus your breathing into your hands, allowing your spasm to soften. With focused breathing, you will soon find your discomfort has decreased. You will have more confidence in your ability to bring healing and comfort to your body.

Painful Gas

After surgery for a Cesarean section, it is important to provide gentle movement and pressure on the abdominal contents to reduce the pain of gas cramps. Usually, the peak of this discomfort is reached on the second or third day after surgery. Simple pelvic floor exercises can be performed in the hospital to help you deal with any pain and discomfort.

GENTLE POST-CESAREAN SECTION EXERCISES

Most of the following exercises can be performed while lying in bed. They should be done gently and easily.

Pelvic Rocking

Benefits

- Stimulates the inner abdominal area, thereby improving digestion and elimination
- Reduces tension from the neck and spine
- Is an excellent energizer

Directions

1. Lie flat on your back.

2. Using your abdominal and buttocks muscles, gently rock your pelvis back and forth.
3. Do this exercise many times during the day.

Cautions and Comments

- After a Cesarean section, your back may be painful. Make sure you rock very slowly and gently.

Ankle and Foot Stretch

Benefits

- Strengthens and stretches ankle and foot muscles: extensor pollicus and digitorum longi, anterior tibialis, posterior tibialis, flexor digitorum longus, peroneus longus and brevis
- Improves circulation in your legs and feet, which prevents blood clots from forming

Directions

1. Lie comfortably with your legs straight out and together.
2. Point and flex your feet at the ankles. Do this 8 times.
3. Separate your legs and circle each foot 8 times to the right and then 8 times to the left.

Cautions and Comments

- These two movements will improve your leg circulation, especially if you are in bed most of the day.

Leg Slides

Benefits

- Gently stretches the hamstring muscles
- Helps close the separation between the recti (abdominal) muscles (see page 120)
- Strengthens abdominalis, iliopsoas, gastrocnemius, and soleus muscle groups; quadriceps; anterior tibialis, extensor digitorum, and hallucis longus muscles

Directions

1. Lying down with your knees bent, push your lower back into the bed tilting your pelvis. Put one hand under your back and check that you are holding a pelvic tilt.
2. Take an Abdominal Breath (page 17) and blow out while rocking your pelvis. Rock your pelvis by tightening your tummy and tucking your buttocks muscles under. The back of your waist should be firmly pressed into the bed.
3. Focus on keeping your lower back on the bed without arching up, and slide your legs (one at a time) away from your buttocks (Figure 9.8).
4. Take an Abdominal Breath between leg slides.
5. Repeat 5 times for each leg.
6. After doing this exercise for 3-5 days, slide both feet down together and back up again. Do this 6-12 times.

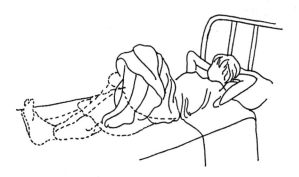

Figure 9.8   Leg Slides

Cautions and Comments

- Initially you may not be able to slide both feet together for more than a few inches, therefore you should start this exercise using one leg at a time.
- Your back arches up when you have weak abdominal muscles. Gradually control and strength will improve so that you will be able to slide down and return without lifting your lower back from the bed.

Partial Curl-Ups

Benefits

- Strengthens iliopsoas muscle group, rectus abdominalis and oblique abdominalis, pectoral muscles, latissimus dorsi, anterior cervical muscles
- Stretches the cervical, thoracic, and lumbosacral erector spinae, glutei muscles, upper trapezius

Directions

1. Lie down with your knees bent and take an Abdominal Breath (page 17).
2. Blowing out, tilt your pelvis up by pulling in your tummy muscles, squeezing your buttocks together, and dropping your chin on your chest.
3. Lift your head and shoulders as high as you can. Stretch your hands towards your feet. Hold this position while breathing normally for 5 counts, and then lower yourself back down slowly (Figure 9.9).
4. Start with 5 Partial Curl-Ups and work up to 10.

5. Once you can easily do 10 Partial Curl-Ups, try doing them with your hands behind your head or crossed over your chest.

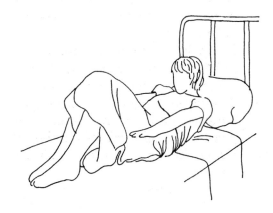

Figure 9.9   Partial Curl-Up

Cautions and Comments

- Be sure to tilt your pelvis up and pull in on your abdominal muscles. This position protects your back and will flatten your tummy much faster.

The Bridge

Benefits

- Helps strengthen the spine
- Relieves lower-back pain
- Relieves neck strain and tension
- Tones and stimulates the central nervous system
- Stretches iliopsoas muscle groups, pectoral muscle groups
- Strengthens thoracic and lumbar erector spinae, gluteals, hamstrings, and soleus muscles

Directions

1. Lie on your back with your knees bent and take an Abdominal Breath (page 17).
2. While blowing out the breath, tilt your pelvis up by pulling in your abdominal muscles.
3. Slowly lift your buttocks and back to form a straight line from your shoulders to your knees (Figure 9.10).
4. Breathe normally as you contract your buttocks and abdominal muscles, then twist to the right and then to the left.
5. Slowly lift your back to the starting postion.
6. Repeat 5 times.

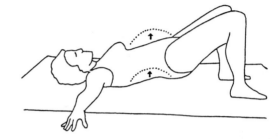

Figure 9.10   The Bridge

Cautions and Comments

- Lower your spine back down very slowly and carefully, instead of plopping down.
- As a variation, try going up on your toes when you are in the bridge position.

Abdominal Breaths

See page 17 for complete instructions.

Shoulder Circles and Shrugs

See page 126 for complete instructions.

Shoulder Stretch-Backs

See page 126 for complete instructions.

AN ENCOURAGING WORD TO ALL NEW MOTHERS

Healing after the birth of your baby depends upon your own personal birth experience. Three weeks after a vaginal birth or six weeks after a Cesarean birth you should be able to go on to Step #2 of the Positive Parenting Fitness program, found in the following chapter. Step #2 includes the Basic Eight and the Sun and Moon Salutes. These special stretching exercises should be practiced for at least one month before going on to Step #3. Each new mother takes a different time to heal, but please remember that rushing into strenuous exercises too soon after giving birth can result in possible injury. Motherhood takes patience with your baby as well as with your body.

CHAPTER TEN

Step 2
The Basic Eight and the
Sun and Moon Salutes

Step #2 of the Positive Parenting Fitness program includes special stretching exercises that are designed to encourage your body back into shape gently and naturally. Practicing the Basic Eight exercises in conjunction with the Sun and Moon Salutes will effectively help you get your body back into shape. These exercises also promote healing.

Before going into the exercises in Step #2, please take a few minutes and read through the following Do's and Don'ts. If you follow these simple guidelines, you will look forward to your practice sessions. Declare 20-30 minutes a day as your private time. Take the phone off the hook; tune out the world for a short time. You will find that both you and your baby will emerge from this time feeling refreshed and renewed.

GUIDELINES FOR
STRETCHING EXERCISES

- *Do* check with your health-care provider before starting any exercise program.
- *Do* make your practice time a play time for you and your baby.
- *Do* try to be consistent in the amount of time you practice—20-30 minutes a day is fine.
- *Do* practice on a comfortable exercise mat.
- *Do* wear loose, comfortable clothing. Leotards are not necessary.
- *Do* move slowly and gracefully from one exercise to another.
- *Do* take a 2:8:4 Breath (page 18) between exercises.
- *Do* keep your mind on what you are doing and on your baby as you move and stretch.
- *Do* end your practice sessions with several Abdominal Breaths (page 17) and the Total Relaxation Exercise (page 121).

- *Don't* practice if you feel pain. If you find yourself in pain, stop! Re-evaluate the exercise, your position, and/or your approach. *Do not* accept pain as a natural consequence of exercise. Pain is a warning to stop!
- *Don't* rush through a practice session.
- *Don't* practice in a poorly ventilated room.
- *Don't* practice right after eating. Wait an hour or two.
- *Don't* hold an exercise beyond the comfort level. When an exercise becomes uncomfortable, that is your signal to stop and breathe.
- *Don't* practice when you are ill. Use deep-breathing or relaxation exercises only.
- *Don't* mentally criticize yourself when you are practicing.
- *Don't* practice the more difficult exercises without some preliminary warm-ups.
- *Don't* concentrate on a series of exercises for only one area of the body. Try to make each session balanced by stretching and moving in all directions.

The Basic Eight

Time is often in short supply when a new baby enters your life. The Basic Eight exercise series was developed with this very crucial fact in mind. It contains a variety of highly effective, yet easy-to-learn exercises, which will quickly tone, tighten, and renew your body while calming and quieting your mind. If you find only a few spare moments during the day, these exercises are the best. Once you have done them for a short while, you will begin to feel the logic of their order and the resulting benefits.

These particular exercises were chosen for the Basic Eight because they produce the best results in the least amount of time. My Positive Parenting Fitness classes always practice these exercises in conjunction with the Sun and Moon Salutes (beginning on page 154) for a complete workout in the early weeks postpartum.

You will find that as you work with these exercises you will be able to hold each position for longer periods of time as your body becomes more supple.

1.   Rock and Rolls

Benefits

- Warms and limbers the spine, therefore an excellent warm-up exercise
- Reduces tension from the neck and spine
- Is an excellent energizer
- Stimulates the inner abdominal area, thereby improving digestion and elimination
- Strengthens the abdominal muscles
- Stretches cervical, thoracic, and lumbar erector spinae muscle groups, hip rotators, perineal muscles, hip adduc-

tors, ankle/toe extensors, and dorsi flexors

• Strengthens anterior neck muscles, pectorals, elbow flexors, latissimus dorsi, gluteals, hip adductors

Directions for Variation I

1. Sit in a comfortable, cross-legged position and take 1-2 Abdominal Breaths (page 17).
2. Place your left hand on your right toes and your right hand on your left toes.

Holding your feet tightly (Figure 10.1A), slowly begin to roll backward (Figure 10.1B). It is often helpful to bend your head toward your toes for the first Rock and Roll.

3. Once you roll backward, use the force of this movement to return to your starting position.
4. Continue to roll backward and forward 5-6 times, breathing normally, until your spine feels warm and tingly. You will notice an easy rhythm as you rock.

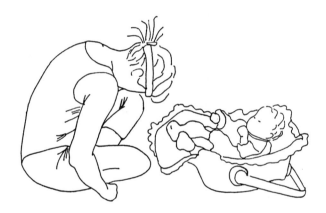

A. STARTING POSITION

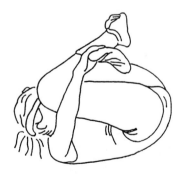
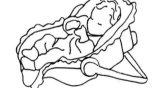

B. ROLLING BACKWARD

Figure 10.1   Rock and Rolls: Variation I

Directions for Variation II

1. Sit with your knees bent and your hands clasped around your knees (Figure 10.2A); your ankles can be crossed or uncrossed. Take 1-2 Abdominal Breaths (page 17).
2. Bend your head forward close to your knees and proceed to roll backward (Figure 10.2B).
3. Once you roll backward, use the force of this movement to return you to your starting position.
4. Continue to roll backward and forward 5-6 times, breathing normally, until your spine feels warm and tingly. You will notice an easy rhythm as you rock.

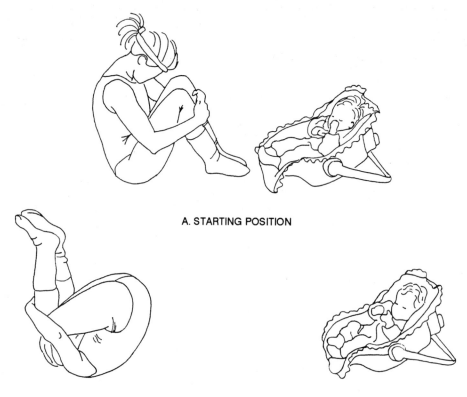

A. STARTING POSITION

B. ROLLING BACKWARD

Figure 10.2   Rock and Rolls: Variation II

Cautions and Comments

• Practice on a soft mat with plenty of padding.
• Before beginning this exercise, make sure the area around you is clear; you don't want to hit anything when rolling backward.
• If you prefer, you can begin this exercise on your back and roll up into a sitting position.
• It is important to have a rounded spine for this exercise, so try to keep your head close to your knees in either of the variations.
• Rock and Rolls are excellent for removing any kinks from the spine.

2.   Abdominal Lift

Benefits

- Tightens and firms the abdominal muscles
- Stimulates the inner abdominal area, thereby improving digestion and elimination
- Helps reduce the waistline
- Stretches thoracic and lumbar erector spinae
- Strengthens all divisions of the abdominalis muscle group (rectus, obliques, transversus) and gluteal muscles

Directions for Variation I: Cat Position

1. Assume a hands and knees position with your weight evenly distributed.
2. Take a deep breath and exhale completely. Now exhale a bit more—there is always more to exhale. *Do not inhale again until this exercise is completed.*
3. Relax your stomach and suck your tummy muscles in and upward behind your rib cage (Figure 10.3). This will give you a tight feeling in your throat and cause a hollow in the stomach area if practiced correctly. Try to pull your tummy muscles even higher.
4. Hold for 5-30 seconds, release the muscles, and inhale.
5. Repeat 3-5 times, being sure to take several Abdominal Breaths (page 17) between contractions.

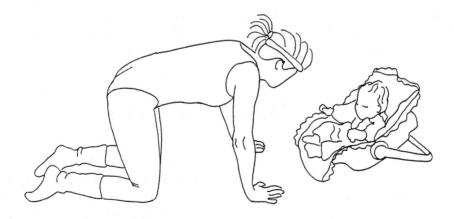

Figure 10.3   Abdominal Lift: Cat Position

Directions for Variation II:
Standing Position

1. Stand up straight with your feet shoulder distance apart. Bend your knees and place your hands on your thighs just above or on the side of your knees.
2. Follow directions 2-5 of Variation I.

Directions for Variation III:
Sitting Position

1. Sit in a comfortable cross-legged position. Place your hands on your knees (Figure 10.4).
2. Follow directions 2-5 of Variation I.

Cautions and Comments

*   This exercise should always be practiced on an empty stomach
*   If you are exhaling after you have released the lift, you are not doing this exercise correctly.
*   Bringing your chin to your chest will help you hold your breath.
*   Take at least 20 seconds to exhale be-

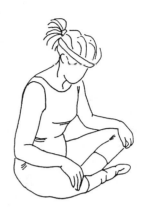

Figure 10.4   Abdominal Lift: Sitting Position

fore you pull in and up on your tummy.
*   If you are suffering from constipation, drink a glass of warm water that contains the juice of one freshly squeezed lemon. Wait 5 minutes and do 5-6 Abdominal Lifts. Then stay close to the bathroom!
*   Practice Abdominal Lifts while feeding your baby.
*   Once you have mastered the three variations, try holding the lift while moving your outer abdominal muscles in and out.

3.   Sitting Spinal Twist

Benefits

*   Helps tighten the waistline
*   Keeps the spine limber
*   Twisting movement tones the nervous system and helps calm jangled nerves
*   Relieves tension in the neck and shoulders; realigns the vertebrae
*   Is an excellent energizer
*   Stretches and strengthens cervical spine rotators (on same side as twist), pectoral muscle groups, biceps brachii, lateral trunk muscles, hip rotators, iliotibial band, gluteals. Each stretch position will affect the opposite musculature, strengthening one side while stretching the other.

Directions

1. Sit up straight in a comfortable cross-legged position with your baby on your lap.
2. Stretch your left arm and place your left hand on your right knee.
3. Stretch your right arm as far behind you as you can (Figure 10.5A), and place your right hand on the floor.
4. Turn your head and look over your right shoulder (Figure 10.5B).
5. Relax your shoulders, facial muscles, and your extended arm, and twist a bit further.
6. Hold for 10-20 seconds or longer.
7. Return to the starting position, take 1-2 Abdominal Breaths (page 17), and repeat on the other side.
8. Do this exercise 2 times on each side.

Cautions and Comments

- Twisting from one side to the other tones the nervous system and helps calm jangled nerves.
- Try keeping the hand that is behind you as close to you as is comfortable. This will give you a better twist.
- To increase the twist, you can bend the arm that is in front of you and stretch your forward shoulder closer to the opposite knee.
- You can play peek-a-boo with your baby while doing this exercise.

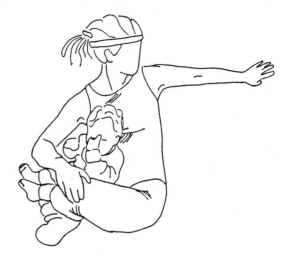

A. STRETCHING YOUR ARM BACK

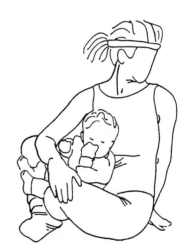

B. LOOKING OVER YOUR SHOULDER

Figure 10.5 Sitting Spinal Twist

4.   The Bridge with Baby

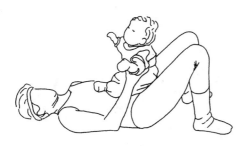

A. STARTING POSITION

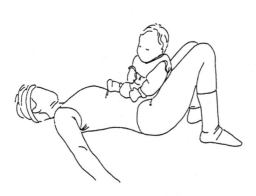

B. RAISING YOUR LOWER BACK

Figure 10.6   Pelvic Rock

Benefits

- Tones, trims, and firms the thighs and buttocks
- Helps strengthen the spine and keep it supple
- Relieves lower-back pain
- Helps make the thighs and hips more shapely
- Relieves neck strain and tension
- Tones and stimulates the central nervous system
- Stretches iliopsoas muscle groups, pectoral muscle groups
- Strengthens thoracic and lumbar erector spinae, gluteals, hamstrings, and soleus muscles

Directions for Pelvic Rock

It is very important to warm-up your lower back *before* doing the Bridge. The Pelvic Rock is the perfect exercise for this.

1.   Lie on your back with your knees bent and your feet flat on the floor about 8 inches apart. Place your baby in a sitting or lying-down position on your tummy (Figure 10.6A).
2.   Take 1-2 Abdominal Breaths (page 17).
3.   Exhale and flatten lower spine to mat.
4.   Inhale and raise your lower back off the mat as high as you can, giving your baby a ride (Figure 10.6B). Make sure your buttocks remain on the mat.
5.   Repeat 4-5 times.

Directions for the Bridge with Baby

1. When your lower back is warmed up and ready to be stretched, hold on to your baby underneath the arms.
2. Slowly raise the middle section of your body and the baby as high in the air as you can (Figure 10.7A). Hold for 5-15 seconds.
3. Now shift your weight to your right leg, and stretch your left leg up into the air (Figure 10.7B). Hold for 5-30 seconds, then repeat on the other side.
4. Slowly roll your spine back down to the mat with control.
5. Take 1-2 Abdominal Breaths (page 17) and repeat the steps once more.

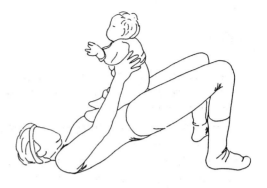

A. RAISING MID-SECTION HIGH IN THE AIR

Cautions and Comments

- Lower your spine to the mat slowly and carefully instead of plopping down.
- This exercise is easy to do while your baby is light; when he becomes a bit heavier, this exercise will become a more strenuous workout for your legs and spine.
- Babies love this routine; it should be a part of your daily practice session.
- As a variation, try going up on your toes when in the bridge position.
- You can follow this exercise with a Lower-Back Massage with Baby (page 244).

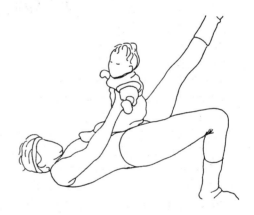

B. STRETCHING LEG INTO THE AIR

Figure 10.7 The Bridge with Baby

5.   The Shoulderstand

Benefits

- Because it oxygenates the brain, spine, and pelvic area, the Shoulderstand is a marvelous rejuvenator.
- Tones, shapes, and energizes the legs, buttocks, and hips
- Tones the central nervous system, which helps eliminate insomnia, tension, and nervous energy
- Massages inner organs, which helps regulate the digestive process to help rid toxins from the body
- Highly beneficial for eliminating menstrual cramps, hemorrhoids, and urinary tract disorders
- Helps relieve aching legs due to varicose veins
- Revitalizes the sex glands and organs, which should give a boost to your sexual drive
- Stretches the spine while strengthening the muscles of the back, legs, neck, shoulders, and abdomen.
- Stretches cervical, thoracic, and lumbar erector spinae; pectoral muscles, hamstrings
- Strengthens the erector spinae muscle groups, abdominals, quadriceps, chest and scapular muscles, gluteals, perineal muscles

Directions for Preparing Your Lower Back

1. Lie flat on your back on top of your mat.
2. Place a thin folded blanket or a piece of foam rubber under your shoulders. Your head should be off this blanket completely, resting comfortably on the mat.
3. Place your baby beside you if you have practiced this exercise before but a fair distance away if this is your first time.
4. Bring your knees to your chest and wrap your arms around them (Figure 10.8).
5. Gently rock from side to side for 1-2 minutes.

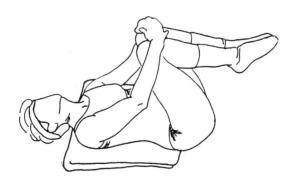

Figure 10.8   Preparing Back for Shoulderstands

**Directions for Variation I:
Full Shoulderstand**

1. Straighten out your legs and lie with your arms close to your body, palms facing down.

2. Take 1-2 Abdominal Breaths (page 17).

3. Close your eyes and imagine that your body is lighter than air. Visualize your legs being lifted off the mat, then your buttocks, and finally your back. (This imaginary concentration will help you practice a smoother, more graceful shoulderstand.)

4. Now bring your knees to your chest, keeping your lower back as flat as possible (Figure 10.9A). Breathe normally as you straighten your legs into the air (Figure 10.9B).

5. When your legs are perpendicular, press your hands against the mat and raise your lower back and buttocks off the mat (Figure 10.9C).

6. Once your legs, buttocks, and back are in the air, bend your arms at the elbows and brace your back at the bottom of your waist with your hands for better support. Your legs will be hanging over your head at this point in a Half Shoulderstand (Figure 10.9D).

7. Once you have gotten your balance, begin to straighten your legs up in the air. Try to get your body as straight as possible (Figure 10.9E).

8. When in a Half or a Full Shoulderstand, make circles with your ankles to relax your feet. Circle three times in each direction.

9. Now, become perfectly still. Close your eyes and hold the shoulderstand while you concentrate on relaxing. Mentally tell your body:

   • Legs, relax more. (You can bend your knees slightly.)

   • Buttocks, relax and become more limp.

   • Shoulders, relax more. (Feel the weight of your body evenly distributed on your shoulders.)

   • Spine, relax more.

   Feel the tiredness drain from your legs and body as you continue to relax, retaining an inverted position.

10. Hold this position for 15-60 seconds.

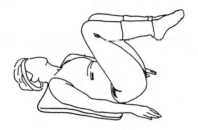

A. BRINGING KNEES TO CHEST

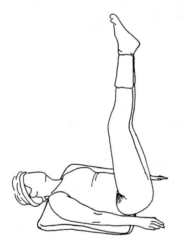

B. STRAIGHTENING LEGS INTO AIR

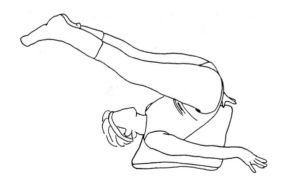

C. RAISING BUTTOCKS OFF MAT

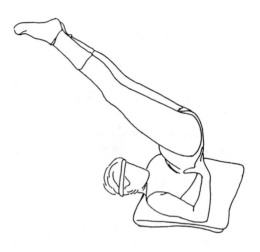

D. SUPPORTING BACK IN HALF SHOULDERSTAND

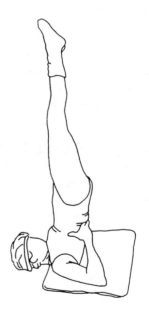

E. THE FULL SHOULDERSTAND

Figure 10.9   Steps for a Full Shoulderstand

Directions for
Coming Out of the Shoulderstand

1. When coming out of the Shoulderstand, remember to *use control.* Bend your knees (Figure 10.10A) and flatten your arms on the mat, palms down.
2. Press on your hands as you *slowly* begin to lower your back to the mat one vertebra at a time (Figure 10.10B).
3. Look behind you as you unroll. This will help keep your spine on the mat and will help you unroll correctly.
4. Once your buttocks are on the mat, take 1-2 Abdominal Breaths (page 17) and then slowly lower your legs. Take at least 15 seconds to get them all the way down. Try to keep your lower back flat as you lower your legs to the mat. *If you have separated recti muscles (page 120), bend your knees directly onto your chest and roll from side to side a few times before straightening your legs back to the mat.*
5. Once you are flat on the mat, take 3-4 Abdominal Breaths, then move your head from side to side to release any tension in your neck.
6. Bring your knees to your chest and wrap your arms around them. Then bring your head to your knees and rock from side to side (Figure 10.10C). This will massage your lower back.
7. Flatten yourself out, take several more Abdominal Breaths, and relax (Figure 10.10D).

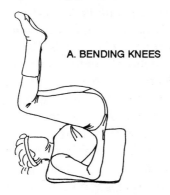

A. BENDING KNEES

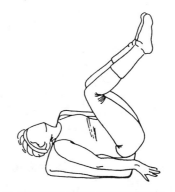

C. ROCKING FROM SIDE TO SIDE

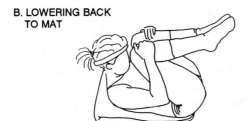

B. LOWERING BACK TO MAT

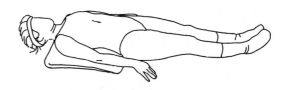

D. FLATTENING OUT

Figure 10.10 Steps for Coming Out of a Shoulderstand

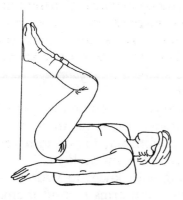

A. PLACING FEET ON WALL

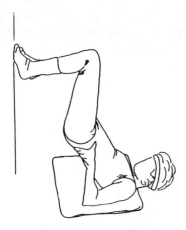

B. LIFTING HIPS AND BUTTOCKS

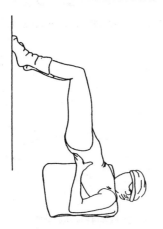

C. WALKING UP WALL

Figure 10.11   Steps for a Wall
                          Shoulderstand

Directions for Variation II:
Wall Shoulderstand

1. While lying on your back, place your feet on a wall (Figure 10.11A).
2. Press into the wall and slowly lift your hips and buttocks into the air (Figure 10.11B).
3. Walk up the wall as far as you can. Breathe normally while holding this position for 30-60 seconds (Figure 10.11C).
4. Slowly lower yourself to the mat, roll over onto your side, and relax.

Cautions and Comments

- *Women with high blood pressure should always have medical consent before practicing shoulderstands.*
- Practice shoulderstands *only* after your lochia flow has stopped.
- The thin blanket placed under your shoulders will protect your neck muscles and vertebrae.
- The Wall Shoulderstand is a good place to start for those new mothers who do not have good control over their abdominal muscles (especially for those who have had a Cesarean delivery).
- It is advisable to practice the Half or Wall Shoulderstand until your spine is strong enough to hold your legs. As your back grows stronger, move your legs higher into the air. One day you will find them straight up!
- Practicing in the early morning may be difficult because of morning stiffness. Wait until later in the day.
- You may have difficulty breathing when in a Half or Full Shoulderstand. Correct blanket placement should eliminate the problem. Once your body

is accustomed to this inverted position, these feelings will pass.

- Place your shoulders as close together as possible. This maximizes body support.
- It is not advisable to hold your breath while doing shoulderstands.
- You may feel dizzy or a bit lightheaded when first practicing this posture. This is caused by an increased flow of blood to the brain. In time and with practice these symptoms will pass.
- If you are suffering from postpartum hemorrhoids, practicing the Squeeze (page 122) while doing a Full or Half Shoulderstand is helpful for speedy healing. Remember to cross your feet at the ankles before contracting your buttocks muscles (Figure 10.12) and hold for a count of 5.

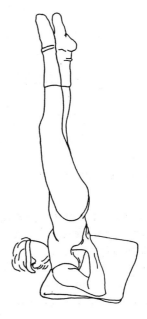

Figure 10.12   "The Squeeze" While in a Full Shoulderstand

6.   The Fish

Benefits

- Tones and gently shapes the buttocks
- Is helpful for eliminating respiratory problems, including asthma
- Helps make the neck and upper back supple and flexible.
- Is helpful for eliminating postpartum hemorrhoids
- Improves blood flow to the head, thereby energizing the body
- Develops the chest and bustline
- Strengthens the spine while releasing tensions
- Stretches abdominalis muscle group, pectoral muscle group, anterior neck muscles (sternocleidomastoid)
- Strengthens cervical, thoracic, and lumbar erector spinae, gluteals, perineal muscles

Directions

1. Lie flat on your back and place your hands, palms down, under your thighs. Push down on your elbows and slowly arch your back. This will raise your chest up into the air.

2. Drop your head back letting it touch the floor. You will feel some pressure or weight on the top of your head, at the base of your spine, and in the buttocks area. The brunt of your weight should be on your buttocks. (Figure 10.13).

3. While breathing normally, relax your legs and feet as you hold this position for 5-30 seconds.

4. Flatten out when you begin to feel uncomfortable, perform 1-2 Abdominal Breaths (page 17), and relax.

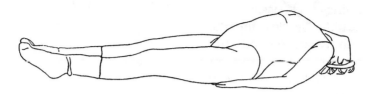

Figure 10.13   The Fish

Cautions and Comments

- This complementary posture should always be practiced when doing shoulderstands (page 144).
- Once you become used to this posture, you will find it easier to maintain normal breathing because your chest area is opened.
- Keep your legs and feet relaxed. It will increase the benefits of this exercise.
- Once in this posture, try to raise your chest up a bit higher in order to maximize the stretch to the spine.

7.   The Universal Pose

Benefits

- Stretches and strengthens opposite side cervical erector spinae and pectoral muscle groups, lateral flank and trunk muscles (quadratus lumborum, obliques), hip rotators, gluteals, iliotibial band, thoracic and lumbar erector spinae
- Loosens, relaxes, and tones the lower back
- Strengthens the spine while keeping it supple
- Tones the shoulders, legs, thighs, and buttocks
- Relieves lower backache

Directions

1. Lie on your back and bend your right leg so that your foot is next to the inside of your left knee.
2. Now, move your hips about 1 inch to the right, and place your left hand on your right knee (Figure 10.14A).
3. Cross your right knee over your left leg and press it into the mat while extending your right arm out to the side. Turn your head to the right (Figure 10.14B).
4. Keep your arms and shoulders as comfortably close to the mat as you can.
5. Hold this posture for 30 seconds to 1 minute as you consciously relax your shoulders, hips, and legs. Breathe normally.
6. Return to the starting position, take 1-2 Abdominal Breaths (page 17), and repeat on the other side.

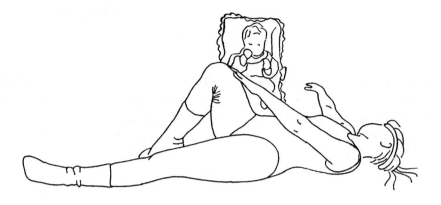

A. STARTING POSITION

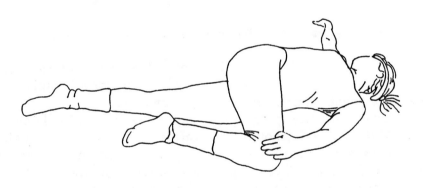

B. FINAL POSITION

Figure 10.14   The Universal Pose

Cautions and Comments

• You may hear the bones in your back crack as you practice this exercise. Don't be alarmed. You are merely breaking up calcium deposits as well as releasing bodily tension and tiredness.

• Moving your hips an inch or so (see step 2) helps give you a better stretch.

• Bending your bottom leg a bit may increase comfort.

• If your top leg does not reach the mat, press on it with the opposite hand, but do not force it down.

8. Complete Relaxation

Benefits

- Deeply relaxes the muscles and the nervous system
- Releases stored tensions and anxieties, thereby restoring a peaceful feeling to the body and the mind
- Twenty minutes of Complete Relaxation is equal to two hours of sleep
- Is an energizer
- Helps keep blood pressure within a normal range

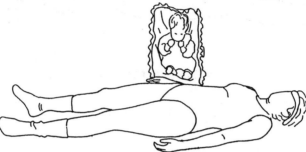

Figure 10.15   The Sponge Position

Directions

1. Lie flat on your back with your arms and legs a comfortable distance apart. See Figure 10.15, the Sponge Position.
2. Take 5 Abdominal Breaths (page 17).
3. Close your eyes and contract all your facial muscles, moving them towards your nose. Hold for 5 seconds, release, and breathe.
4. Next, squeeze your shoulders up around your neck and concentrate on the tightness as you squeeze harder. Hold 5 seconds, release, and breathe.
5. Make fists with your hands and tighten your arms. Tighten harder as you raise your arms a few inches. Hold for 5 seconds, release, and breathe.
6. Squeeze your shoulder blades together, then squeeze a little harder. Hold for 5 seconds, release, and breathe.
7. Contract abdominal and buttock mus-

cles and feel the tightness. Squeeze harder. Hold for 5 seconds, release, and breathe.
8. Tighten your thighs, knees, and calves. Concentrate on the tightness as you squeeze harder. Hold for 5 seconds, release, and breathe.
9. Push your heels away from your body by flexing your toes towards your knees. Feel the tightness. Hold for 5 seconds, release, and breathe.
10. Open your mouth wide and inhale. As you exhale say, "Ah." Repeat 5 times.
11. Now, focus your concentration back on your facial muscles; feel your forehead going limp. Try to relax this area even more.
12. Next, mentally focus on your eyes. Relax your eyes, eye muscles, and eyelids.
13. Feel your jaw and cheek muscles let-

ting go. Feel the looseness. Open your mouth slightly and let your tongue fall back into your mouth. Feel the muscles in your mouth area letting go.

14. Feel your nostrils, ears, and scalp relaxing.
15. Let all expression melt from your face.
16. Relax your neck—the front, sides, and back.
17. Feel your shoulder muscles letting go—the right, the left, and the space between.
18. Feel your upper arms, elbows, and lower arms relaxing.
19. Relax your hands. Start with your thumbs, then relax one finger at a time. Finally, relax your palms.
20. Feel your chest and back going limp.

At this point, the entire top half of your body should be completely loose and relaxed.

21. Next, concentrate on your abdominal muscles. Have them go limp.
22. Feel your buttocks going limp.
23. Focus on your vaginal and anal muscles and let them relax.
24. Concentrate on your thighs, hips, knees, calves, and ankles; feel them going limp.

25. Totally relax your feet and toes.
26. Take a moment or two to check your body for any further tensions. Mentally command any remaining tight spots to go limp and loose.
27. Feel yourself sinking into the mat—let go—give up. Feel a sense of looseness enveloping you.
28. Now, feel any tensions draining out of your body from your fingers and toes. Imagine this flow of tension, tiredness, troubles, fears, anxieties, and aches leaving your body.
29. Keep your breathing at a comfortable rate as you sink into the blissful feeling of complete relaxation.
30. Keep a mental awareness on the pleasurable sensations of your resting, relaxed body for 10-20 minutes.
31. When coming out of the Complete Relaxation exercise, take your time (even if your baby is crying).
32. First, become aware of how your body feels. Focus on your hands and legs, then slowly move your fingers and toes.
33. Gradually begin to stretch and rouse.
34. Stretch up into a sitting position and stretch your body. You should feel revitalized and energized after your practice.

Cautions and Comments

• Directions for the Complete Relaxation exercise, as well as the directions for the other Basic Eight exercises can be found on the *Shape Up With Baby* audio cassette (see page 309).
• Don't be discouraged if it takes a full twenty minutes to get all of your muscles to relax. Keep practicing until your body responds to the mental commands.
• Try not to fall asleep during this relaxation. Rather go into a deep relaxation or a light meditative state with mental clarity.
• Including this relaxation exercise at the end of any stretching session will balance out the session while leaving you without any post-exercise aches.

The Sun and Moon Salutes

The second part of Step #2 of the Positive Parenting Fitness program includes the Sun and Moon Salutes. This series of linked warm-up stretches are designed to work gently but effectively with the healing process that your body goes through approximately four weeks postpartum. If these stretches are practiced slowly, they become a balanced exercise routine that will help limber and tone your body while calming you down.

After pregnancy, some women find it difficult to balance themselves. The following Salutes have been modified to work with your postpartum body. In time, your balance will return. When practicing the Salutes each movement should flow naturally into the next one.

Before you begin, place your baby about a foot or two in front of you on a blanket or in an infant seat. During the exercises, try to maintain eye contact with your child. Play peek-a-boo when doing the backward bends, and talk to or tickle your child as you practice.

The Sun Salute

Benefits

- Is an excellent warm-up routine
- Reduces weight in the tummy and waist area
- Relieves tension and insomnia
- Activates the respiratory and circulatory systems
- Opens the chest area and improves breathing
- Increases energy level while improving circulation
- Is beneficial for eliminating lethargy and depression
- Stretches and strengthens shoulder and scapular muscles (rotator cuff, pectorals, deltoids, serratus anterior); cervical, thoracic, and lumbar erector spinae; hamstrings; quadriceps; iliopsoas, gastrocnemius, and soleus muscle groups

Directions

1.   Stand up straight with your feet about 8 inches apart, facing forward. Place your hands, palms together in a prayer position, with your thumbs resting against your breastbone (Figure 10.16).

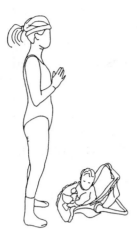

Figure 10.16   Standing Prayer Position

2. Take an Abdominal Breath (page 17) and exhale completely. Use normal breathing throughout the remainder of this series. (Note that inhale and exhale instructions are indicated.)

3. Stretch your arms out in front of your chest and interlock your thumbs (Figure 10.17). Continue moving your arms up until they are stretched toward the ceiling with your upper arms next to your ears.

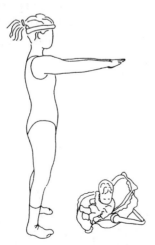

Figure 10.17   Backward Bend
                   Starting Position

4. Relax your knees a bit and push your pelvis forward while carefully bending backward as far as you can (Figure 10.18). Hold this stretch 5-20 seconds. (Inhale)

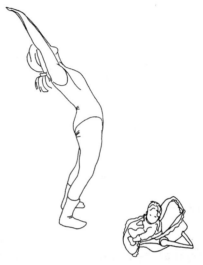

Figure 10.18   Bending Backward

5. Now bring your arms forward and down into a full forward bend while keeping your knees straight. Tickle baby on the way down (Figure 10.19), and then, if you can, place the palms of your hands flat on the mat in line with your feet. If you cannot reach the mat, let your arms dangle towards the

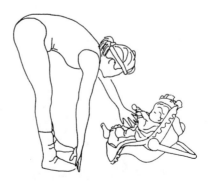

Figure 10.19   Tickling Baby

ground (do not bounce). Release your head and let it hang down (Figure 10.20). Let the weight of your upper body help you get down even lower. Relax in this position as you hold for 5-20 seconds. (Exhale)

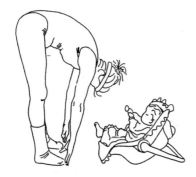

Figure 10.20   Dangling Your Arms

6.   Bend at the knees and slide your right leg back, keeping your right knee and right foot flat on the mat. Your hands should be flat on the mat in line with your left (forward) foot. Reach for the ceiling with your chin. Push your groin area toward the mat. This will cause your back to arch (Figure 10.21). Relax and hold this position for 5-10 seconds. (Inhale)

7.   Next, slide your left foot back next to your right foot. Push your buttocks up into the air while touching your chin to your chest in an Inverted "V" Position (Figure 10.22). Try to get your heels as close to the mat as possible. Don't cheat by moving your feet closer to your head! Hold for 5-20 seconds. (Inhale)

8.   Without moving your hands, bring your

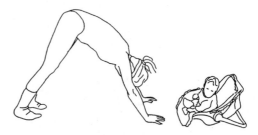

Figure 10.32   Inverted "V" Position

knees down to the mat followed by your hips. Slide your legs back a bit. Raise your head and shoulders while keeping your arms bent. Reach for the ceiling with your chin (feel the stretch in the middle of your back). Straighten out your arms and reach higher with your chin. Keep the lowest part of your abdomen on the mat in this Cobra Position (Figure 10.23). Hold for 5-20 seconds. (Inhale)

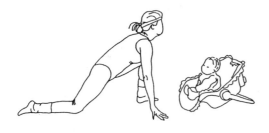

Figure 10.21   Arching Your Back

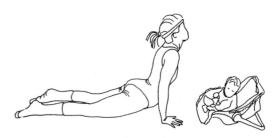

Figure 10.23   Cobra Position

9. Next, return to the Inverted "V" Position by curling your toes under and pushing yourself up from the bottom of your spine until your buttocks is lifted into the air. Bring your chin to your chest and stretch your heels down toward the mat (Figure 10.24). Hold for 5-20 seconds. (Exhale)

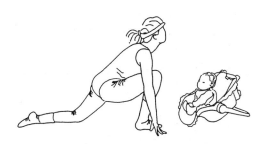

Figure 10.25 Arching Your Back

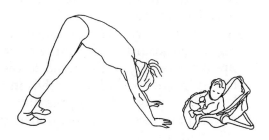

Figure 10.24 Inverted "V" Position

10. Place your knees on the mat and bring your right foot up so that it is between and in line with your hands. Slide your left foot back as far as possible, keeping your left knee and left foot flat. Arch your back by reaching toward the ceiling with your chin while keeping your hands flat on the mat and your groin pushed towards the ground (Figure 10.25). Hold for 5-20 seconds. (Inhale)

11. Bring your left foot forward so that it is in line with your right foot. (Your feet should be about 8 inches apart.) Raise your buttocks so that you are in a Forward Bend (Figure 10.26). Place your palms flat on the floor next to your feet if you can. Hold for 5-20 seconds. (Exhale)

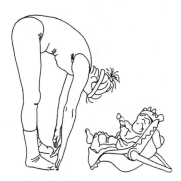

Figure 10.26 Forward Bend

12. Interlock your thumbs and stretch your arms up toward the ceiling until your upper arms are next to your ears. Relax your knees a bit and push your pelvis forward, while carefully bending backward as far as you can (Figure 10.27). Hold for 5-20 seconds. (Inhale)

Cautions and Comments

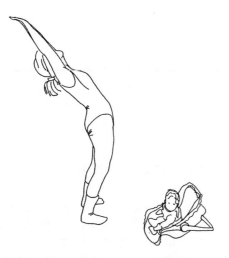

Figure 10.27   Backward Bend

13.   Bring your hands back into the Standing Prayer Position (Figure 10.28) and take 2-3 Abdominal Breaths (page 17).

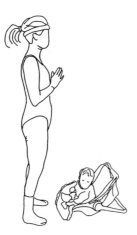

Figure 10.28   Standing Prayer Position

14.   Repeat the steps of the Sun Salute 2-3 times. These steps can also be done more quickly by holding each position for only 1-2 seconds. If you have chosen this quicker version, repeat the steps 5-10 times.

- The Sun Salute *is not recommended* for women with high blood pressure, heart ailments, slipped disks, or lower-back pain.
- Don't be discouraged if you do not look like the model in the drawings when you are in each position. With practice and discipline you will eventually stretch into and perfect each part of this series.
- If you notice any back pain when doing the Backward Bend, simply reach up to the ceiling and proceed to the next step. The joints of your pelvis and lower back may be less supple due to certain pregnancy hormones that may still be in your body.
- If you have an excessive lower-back curvature or if you had lower-back pain during your pregnancy, these extension exercises are not suitable for you. Exercises that *round* your lower back are recommended until you are pain-free. (Refer to Chapter Fourteen, "Exercises Designed to Relieve Backaches.")
- Do not force your body to go beyond its limits. Stretch as far as is comfortable in each direction.
- Practice in front of a window bathed in sunlight. Let the warmth of the sun help your muscles stretch.
- Play peaceful music while practicing. This will help you move more slowly and smoothly. See page 310 for peaceful music cassette titles.
- Interact with your baby by keeping eye and voice contact with him throughout these movements; playing peek-a-boo during the Backward Bends is a fun way to interact.

The Moon Salute

Benefits

- Extremely beneficial for slimming the waist, hips, and thighs
- Is a calming, cooling series
- Releases stored tensions; calms an agitated body and mind
- Strengthens, tones, and stretches the calves and thighs
- Strengthens and revitalizes the spine
- Stretches and opens the chest and shoulder areas
- Is an excellent warm-up series
- Stretches and strengthens primary anterior, lateral, and posterior cervical muscles (sternocleidomastoid, upper trapezius, erector spinae); latissimus dorsi; quadratus lumborum; obliques and rectus abdominalis; pectoral muscle groups; hamstrings; gastrocnemius and soleus muscles

Directions

1. Stand up straight with your feet about 3 feet apart, facing forward.
2. Extend your right arm out to the side, then bring it up until your upper arm is next to your right ear.
3. Slide your left arm down your left leg as you stretch your right arm straight out and parallel to the floor (Figure 10.29). Make sure your back is straight, not twisted.
4. Relax your neck for increased comfort, then maximize this stretch by extending your right arm more. Hold this position for 5-30 seconds while relaxing into the stretch.
5. Roll up slowly, then gently lower your right arm to your side.
6. Take 1-2 Abdominal Breaths (page 17) and repeat on the left side.
7. Next, extend your right arm out to the side again and bring it up until your upper arm is next to your right ear.

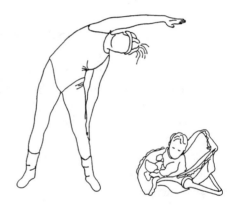

Figure 10.29 Side Stretch with Straight Arm

Now, bend your arm and bring your right hand over your head. Turn your head to the right and face your inner elbow.

8. Holding that position, slide your left arm down your left leg as far as you can (Figure 10.30). Keep your back straight and make sure your arm does not fall in front of you. Relax into the stretch and hold for 5-30 seconds.
9. Take 1-2 Abdominal Breaths (page 17) and repeat on the left side.

12. Slowly roll up and continue moving forward into a complete Forward Bend (Figure 10.32). Relax into the stretch and hold for 5-30 seconds.

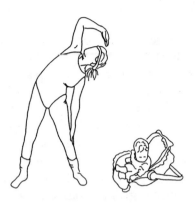

Figure 10.30   Side Stretch with Bent Arm

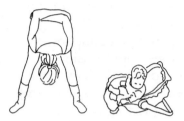

Figure 10.32   Forward Bend

10. Stand up straight and fold your arms behind your back. (Place your right hand on your left elbow or upper arm and your left hand on your right elbow or upper arm. The higher you place your hands, the greater the shoulder stretch.)

11. Stretch your chin up toward the ceiling and slowly bend back as far as you can (Figure 10.31). Relax into the stretch and hold for 5-30 seconds.

13. Slowly roll up into a standing position and take 1-2 Abdominal Breaths (page 17).

14. Keeping your arms folded behind you, turn your left foot on a 90° angle and move your right foot forward about 6 inches for better balance. Now turn your upper body toward your left leg (don't lock your knees) and stretch your chin out to the left as you stretch your head down toward your knee (Figure 10.33) in a thigh stretch.

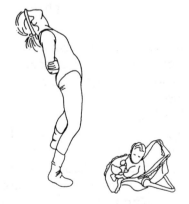

Figure 10.31   Backward Bend

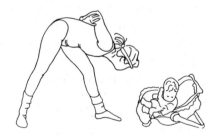

Figure 10.33   Thigh Stretch

15. Once you have stretched down as far as you can, relax your neck and try to bring your forehead to your knee. Hold this position for 5-30 seconds while relaxing into the stretch. Pay special attention to relaxing the area behind your knees.
16. Slowly roll up, stretching your chin forward as you return to a standing position.
17. Take 1-2 Abdominal Breaths (page 17) and repeat on the other side.
18. Repeat the steps of the Moon Salute 3-4 times. As with the Sun Salute, these steps can be done more quickly by holding each position for only 1-2 seconds. If you choose the quicker version, repeat the steps 5-10 times.

Cautions and Comments

- The Moon Salute *is not recommended* for women with high blood pressure, heart ailments, slipped disks, or lower-back pain.
- Do not hold any one movement too long as this can result in soreness.
- If you have trouble with balance during the thigh stretch, move your back foot (the one you are *not* stretching) forward a bit.
- The more you separate your feet, the greater the depth of each stretch.
- Try to move very slowly, smoothly, and gracefully from one step of the series to the next.

Step #2 of the Positive Parenting Fitness program will help make your body feel and look better while it calms your mind. The Basic Eight and the Sun and Moon Salutes help speed the healing process inside your body while toning it on the outside. In time, you will come to enjoy the steady flow of the movements and the revitalizing benefits they bring.

CHAPTER ELEVEN
Step 3
Your Complete
Body Workout

For approximately six months after you've had your baby, your joints will be more flexible and less secure. Therefore, it may take up to six months or more for your body to revert back to normal. Step #3 of the Positive Parenting Fitness program takes this into consideration and offers a complete body workout.

According to many exercise physiologists, a proper, safe, and effective workout combines three separate components that are practiced in a proper sequence. The first component is the initial *warm-up stage* that includes two steps: rhythmic limbering and static stretches. These warm-ups are needed to raise your body's core temperature just slightly. This is important in preparing your body for the work that lies ahead. The second major component of a proper body workout includes *low-impact aerobics.* This part of the workout works your muscles while raising your heart rate. Special aerobic guidelines and procedures will be presented later in this chapter. Finally, a *cool-down period* is mandatory at the end of any effective workout in order to gradually decrease your heart rate until it is back to its normal state. It also prevents the pooling of blood in your legs.

Warm-Ups

RHYTHMIC LIMBERING

The warm-up stage of your complete body workout should begin with rhythmic limbering. The simple movements involved warm up your muscles while increasing the blood flow to your arms and legs. Rhythmic limbering prepares your body for the second half of the warm-ups: the static stretches.

Rhythmic Limbering Movements

Benefits

- Increases flexibility of tendons and ligaments
- Increases core body temperature
- Increases range of motion
- Increases blood flow to extremities

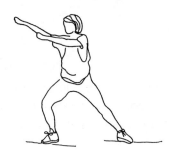

Figure 11.1   Arm Swings

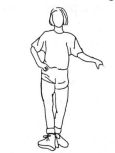

Figure 11.2   Low Kicks

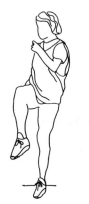

Figure 11.3   Low Knee Lifts

Directions for Arm Swings

1. Stand with your feet about 12 inches apart, pointing slightly outward.
2. Bend your right knee slightly as you swing both arms out to the right (Figure 11.1).
3. Now, with a sweeping motion, swing your arms back out to the left reversing your leg positions.
4. Swing left and right 8 times.

Directions for Low Kicks

5. Now lean all your weight on your left leg and slowly kick your right leg out in front of you 8 times (Figure 11.2). Your arms should be swinging freely.
6. Repeat 8 times with the left leg.

Directions for Low Knee Lifts

7. Skip in place. Bend and raise your right knee up into the air as your left hand swings upward (Figure 11.3).
8. Repeat, alternating on each side, 8 times.

Cautions and Comments

- These movements should be free and easy and fun to do!
- They prepare your body for harder movements and work
- All movements should be done with loose joints, especially your knees.
- *Do not lock your knees or your elbows!*

STATIC STRETCHES

Stretching helps relieve tension and restore flexibility to your muscles and joints while encouraging a free, revitalized flow of blood to your muscles as they relax. Some forms of stretching affect various parts of the body (see Basic Eight exercises beginning on page 136), while other forms, known as static stretches, concentrate on one specific set of muscles at a time. Static stretches help realign your body's joints and improve your shape and posture. Because they enhance circulation and respiration, they can improve nutrition to your cells and tissues. They also ensure that you relax properly and completely. The static stretching exercises that are part of the Positive Parenting Fitness program are designed to work specific muscle groups, head to toe, in order to get your body properly warmed up and ready to begin a low-impact aerobic workout.

General Benefits

• Enhances range of motion through gradual lengthening of muscles

• Prepares the body for more vigorous exercise

• Helps prevent injury

General Guidelines

1. Stretches should be sustained and static.

2. *Do not bounce!* Bouncing increases the risk of over-stretching your muscles. When you bounce, you may stretch beyond the *stretch reflex* (the point where the stretch begins to feel uncomfortable) and injure yourself.

3. Hold each stretch for 15-30 seconds.

Neck Smiles

Benefits

- Promotes full, pain-free neck motion
- May relieve pain and tension in the neck
- Keeps the neck and shoulders loose and limber
- Encourages the relaxation of facial and jaw muscles—a key to general relaxation
- Helps to relax the entire body, eliminates insomnia, and prevents headaches
- Stretches and strengthens the sternocleidomastoid and trapezius muscle groups

Directions

1. Sit up straight in any comfortable sitting position. Close your eyes, letting your head fall loosely forward with your chin near your chest (Figure 11.4).

2. Now imagine that your lips are drawing an imaginary smile in the space directly in front of you. Keeping your shoulders still, slowly move your chin until it is directly above your right shoulder. Draw an imaginary straight line from your right shoulder to your left shoulder as you move your head slowly over to the left.

3. Once your chin is above the left shoulder, release the muscles in the back of your neck and allow your chin to come down as close to your body as possible. Draw the imaginary curving bottom of the smile as you move your head from left to right.

4. Repeat these movements making 3 smiles, beginning on the right, going across to the left, and returning to the right again. Take about 15 seconds to draw one smile. Be sure your movements are smooth and fluid.

5. Repeat 4 times.

Cautions and Comments

- Your neck may crack and creak. Don't worry—you are not falling apart! This is perfectly normal and helpful for keeping the neck area—a very popular tension spot—loose and limber.
- Practice this exercise during television commercials or whenever you have a spare moment.
- This exercise is especially helpful for women who work in offices and spend much of their time looking down.
- Keep neck and shoulders relaxed.

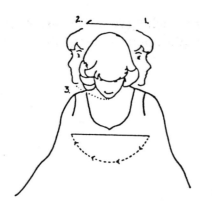

Figure 11.4   Neck Smiles: Various Positions

Shoulder/Upper-Back Stretch

Benefits

- Limbers the shoulders and upper back thereby reducing tension
- Stretches deltoid muscle group; trapezius, teres major and minor, infraspinatus muscles

Directions

1. Keeping your shoulders squared, cross one arm in front of your chest with the elbow bent.
2. Place your free hand on the elbow and gently pull it across your body (Figure 11.5). Hold stretch 15-30 seconds.
3. Repeat with the other arm.

Cautions and Comments

- Do not lock elbows or rotate your waist.
- Keep your shoulders and hips squared.

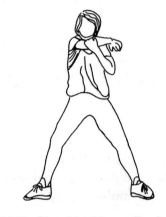

Figure 11.5 Shoulder/Upper-Back Stretch

Tricep Stretch

Benefits

- Strengthens and tones back of arm
- Stretches the tricep muscle

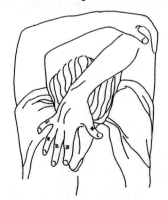

Figure 11.6 Tricep Stretch

Directions

1. With elbow bent, bring one hand up behind your head toward the center of your back.
2. Place your free hand on the bent elbow and gently pull it toward the back of your head (Figure 11.6). Hold stretch 15-30 seconds.
3. Repeat with other arm.

Cautions and Comments

- Do not arch your back.
- Stay in alignment.
- Do not lean to either side.

Side Stretch

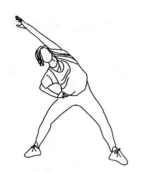

Figure 11.7   Side Stretch

Directions

1. Lean to one side while reaching your arm over your head.
2. Place your free hand on your thigh to support your spine (Figure 11.7). Hold stretch 15-30 seconds.
3. Repeat on the other side.

Benefits

- Lengthens the torso
- Stretches both external and internal oblique muscle groups

Cautions and Comments

- Lean directly over your hip without leaning forward or backward.

Upper-Back Stretch

Benefits

- Releases tension in the upper back and shoulders
- Stretches trapezius, infraspinatus, teres major and minor, rhomboideus major muscles; latissimus dorsi muscles

Cautions and Comments

- Your back should be curved in a "C."
- Your head is an extension of your spine, so make sure it is in a slightly forward position to complete the "C."

Directions

1. Clasp your hands and press them forward (palms away from body) while contracting your abdominals. Press your hips forward (Figure 11.8). Exhale and press 15-30 seconds.
2. Inhale and release.
3. Repeat 4 times.

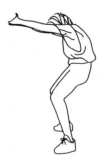

Figure 11.8   Upper-Back Stretch

Hamstring Stretch

Benefits

- Stretches hamstring muscle group
- Reduces tension and stiffness in the arms, neck, and back

Directions

1. Standing up, position one foot in front and one foot behind. Your toes should be facing forward.
2. Keeping your rear heel on the floor, lean forward, bending your front knee (Figure 11.9).
3. Rest both hands on your front thigh to support your spine. Hold stretch 15-30 seconds.
4. Repeat with other leg.

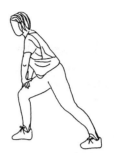

Figure 11.9   Hamstring Stretch

Cautions and Comments

- Keep both heels pressed to the floor.
- Stay in alignment.
- Your front knee should bend directly over your toes. Your front heel should be perpendicular to the toes on your back foot.

Standing Quadriceps Stretch

Benefits

- Tones the front thigh muscles
- Stretches quadricep muscle group

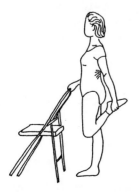

Figure 11.10   Standing Quadriceps Stretch

Directions

1. With your right hand on the back of a chair, hold your left ankle with your left hand and pull the heel in toward your buttocks (Figure 11.10).
2. Lean forward slightly.
3. Hold stretch 15-30 seconds.
4. Repeat with right leg.

Cautions and Comments

- Make sure your ankle and knee are directly behind you.
- Do not arch your back.
- Never lock your knees or elbows.

Standing Calf Stretch

Benefits

- Prevents tightness in lower-leg muscles
- Lengthens and stretches gastrocnemius muscle group

Directions

1. With both hands against a wall, place one foot in front of the other (Figure 11.11).
2. Keep your rear heel down and lean forward bending your front knee. (Your toes should be pointing forward.) Hold stretch 15-30 seconds.
3. Repeat with the other leg.

Cautions and Comments

- Lean your entire body forward as a unit.
- Do not let your rear heel lose contact with the floor.
- Do not hyperextend your lower spine by stretching your buttocks.

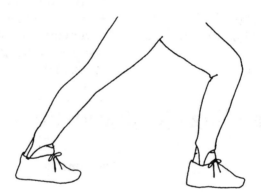

Figure 11.11   Standing Calf Stretch

Straddle Stretch

Benefits

- Lengthens the inner-thigh muscles
- Stretches pectineus, adductor longus and magnus, and gracilis muscles

Directions

1. Sit on the floor with your legs stretched out to your sides, a comfortable distance apart. Slowly lean forward, rotating your hips outward.
2. Place your hands on the floor in front of you to support and stabilize your spine (Figure 11.12).
3. After holding this stretch for 30 seconds, slowly return to the sitting position.

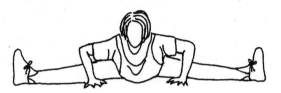

Figure 11.12 Straddle Stretch

Cautions and Comments

- Breathe naturally.
- Do not let your toes or knees roll inward.

Butterfly Stretch

Benefits

- Lengthens the inner-thigh muscles
- Stretches pectineus, the adductor longus, adductor magnus, adductor brevis; gracilis muscle groups

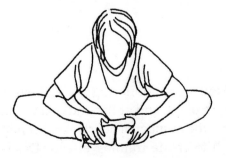

Figure 11.13 Butterfly Stretch

Directions

1. Sit on the floor with the soles of your feet together and your knees out to the sides.
2. Hold onto your ankles and lean forward from your hip (Figure 11.13).
3. Breathe naturally while holding the stretch for 15-30 seconds.
4. Slowly return to the sitting position.

Cautions and Comments

- While bending forward, keep your back flat and your head erect and in line with your spine.

Low-Impact Aerobics

The second main component of a complete body workout, low-impact aerobics, is safe for most postpartum women. According to Diane Milhan, PhD, PT, and Positive Parenting Fitness instructor, when you are ready to begin a cardiovascular training program, the first step should involve low-impact aerobics. Aerobic exercise is important because it strengthens your heart muscle so an increased volume of blood is able to be pumped with fewer contractions. These exercises also burn calories.

The difference between low- and high-impact aerobics relates to the amount of jolting and wear-and-tear to your leg joints when striking the floor. In high-impact aerobics many steps require both feet to be off the ground simultaneously, often allowing only one leg at a time to accept full body weight on landing. In low-impact aerobics, both feet are rarely off the ground simultaneously. Usually one foot, sometimes two, are in constant contact with the floor. Many low-impact aerobic steps are "grounded" versions of steps used in high-impact aerobics. Jumping jacks become heel jacks and jogging becomes marching. In low-impact there is much less percussion and fewer ballistic steps requiring repeated acceptance of your body weight through your leg joints. This, of course, reduces stress to your ankles, knees, and hips. Your back is also relieved of the stress of high-impact movements.

To be most effective, the aerobic segment of your workout should be practiced for twenty minutes a day, two to three times per week. This workout should always be preceded by warm-ups (rhythmic limbering and static stretches) and followed by a cool-down period. Your body needs a chance to recover between aerobic workouts. Vary your workout routines so that you do not practice aerobics two days in a row. On the alternate days you can practice stretching exercises or weight training/Dyna-Band exercises (discussed in Chapter Twelve). However, if scheduling problems should occur, it is safe, but not ideal, to do aerobics for two consecutive days.

TRAINING HEART RATES

Another basic requirement of a good aerobic workout is the monitoring of your heart rate. Heart rates should be monitored before, at the high point, and at the end of a workout. A training heart rate (or target heart rate) represents the number of heartbeats per minute that, when accomplished, is challenging enough to create training effects. Desirable training effects include an increase in fitness as seen in the following signs:

• a lowered resting heart rate (page 174)

• an increase in the amount of blood ejected from the heart with each contraction

• an increase in endurance

• a reduction in the percentage of body fat

• an increase in athletic performance

Training heart rates are determined by several factors including your age, your fitness level, and your current resting heart rate. While exercising below your target heart rate may be beneficial for burning calories, no aerobic fitness will occur. The training heart rate must be demanded by the nature of the exercise and must be maintained for fifteen to twenty minutes at a time.

By establishing a postpartum training heart rate, you will be better able to monitor and then determine the amount of improvement taking place. The formula for establishing your personal training heart rate is found on page 175. The inset on pages 176 and 177 will also be helpful to you when establishing your training heart rate. The important thing to remember is that establishing your own personal training heart rate is considered a helpful guideline, but comfort should always be your main concern.

Finding Your Pulse

Before you can establish your training heart rate you have to be able to monitor your pulse. Before you can do this, you must be able to find your pulse. Your pulse can be felt in the radial artery located in your wrist or in the carotid artery found in your neck.

Do not use your thumb when taking your pulse. As your thumb is also a pulse reference site, you may get confused when counting the beats.

Directions for Finding Radial Pulse

1. Turn your left palm up and place two or three of your right-hand fingertips on the thumb side of your forearm (near the wrist). You will feel a groove between the bone (the radius) and the tendons of the wrist. Inside this groove lies the radial artery.

2. Using gentle touch (too much pressure can cause the artery to move away from your fingertips) you should be able to pick up your pulse.

Directions for Finding Carotid Pulse

1.   Turn your head to the right. On the left side of your neck, you will discover a vertical band of muscles descending from the bone (the mastoid) directly behind your ear.

2.   Slide your fingers down this band, halfway down the neck. Bring your fingertips in front of these muscles. Here you will discover the pulse of the carotid artery.

Establishing a Resting Heart Rate

Establishing your resting heart rate is also necessary before you can formulate your training heart rate. To determine your resting heart rate, you must locate your pulse after a full night's sleep.

1.   Relax in a reclining position (recover from the shock of the alarm clock) for about five minutes.

2.   Locate your pulse as instructed on page 173, and count the number of heartbeats for fifteen seconds.

3.   Multiply the number of heartbeats four times (giving you the number of heartbeats per minute) to determine your resting heart rate.

FORMULA FOR DETERMINING TRAINING HEART-RATE ZONES

Before participating in an exercise program, the individual must determine the desired intensity of the training session. The training heart-rate zone provides the range of acceptable heartbeats during an aerobic exercise session. Several formulas have been established by exercise physiologists to calculate the training heart-rate zone. One of the most convenient formulas, which is also the most individualized, is known as the Heart Reserve Method made popular by Juha Karvonen.

1. This method begins with the number 220, which is considered to be the *theoretical* maximum heart rate at birth. It is believed that this *maximum heart rate* (MHR) decreases by one heartbeat for each year of life. Therefore, to determine your personal maximum heart rate you must subtract your age from 220.

    220 - Age = Personal MHR (maximum heart rate)

2. After establishing your *resting heart rate* (RHR) as explained on page 174, subtract your RHR from your MHR to determine your *heart rate reserve* (HRR). The heart rate reserve number is necessary in determining your personal training zone.

    MHR - RHR = HRR (heart rate reserve)

3. Multiply your HRR by 60 percent and add the resulting number to your RHR. This will establish your *minimum training heart rate*. During a workout session, your heartbeats per minute should not fall below this number.

    HRR x 60% + RHR = *Minimum* training heart rate

4. Multiply your HRR by 80 percent and add the resulting number to your RHR. This will establish your *maximum training heart rate*. During a workout session, your heartbeats per minute should not exceed this number.

    HRR x 80% + RHR = *Maximum* training heart rate

5. This last item is not a step, but as long as I have your attention, it is important to note that the beginning exerciser should start out conservatively. She should exercise at the lower end of her personal heart-rate zone.

Sarah:
Establishing A Training Heart-Rate Zone

By following the procedure for establishing a training heart-rate zone (page 175), let's go through each step of the formula with Sarah, our 32-year-old "sample" mom.

1. Sarah begins with the number 220, which is the *theoretical* maximum heart rate. She then subtracts her age (32) from 220 to arrive at her *personal* maximum heart rate.

    220   *Theoretical* maximum heart rate
    - 32   Sarah's age
    188   Sarah's *personal* maximum heart rate (MHR)

2. Sarah's resting heart rate (RHR) is 72. She arrived at this number by taking her pulse (page 173) after a full night's sleep. After determining how many times her heart beat during 15 seconds, she multiplied this number by 4 and arrived at the number of times her heart beat in one minute (her RHR).

    18   Sarah's number of heartbeats per 15 seconds
    x4   (to establish heartbeats per minute)
    72   Sarah's resting heart rate (RHR)

3. Sarah now subtracts her resting heart rate of 72 (step 2) from her maximum heart rate of 188 (step 1) and arrives at the number 116. This number is her heart rate reserve (HRR).

    188   Sarah's maximum heart rate (step 1)
    - 72   Sarah's resting heart rate (step 2)
    116   Sarah's heart rate reserve (HRR)

4. Now Sarah chooses two multipliers based on the intensity level at which she wishes to work. This intensity level generally ranges from 60 (.6) percent to 80 (.8) percent of one's maximum capacities.

5. Sarah multiplies 116 (heart rate reserve established in step 3) by the *minimum* intensity level of .6, which she has chosen in step 4. She arrives at the number 69.6, which she rounds off to 70.

```
116    Sarah's heart rate reserve (step 3)
x. 6   Minimum intensity-level multiplier (step 4)
 70    (after rounding off 69.6)
```

6. Sarah multiplies 116 (heart rate reserve established in step 3) by the *maximum* intensity level of .8, which she has chosen in step 4. She arrives at the number 92.8, which she rounds off to 93.

```
116    Sarah's heart rate reserve (step 3)
x. 8   Maximum intensity-level multiplier (step 4)
 93    (after rounding off 92.8)
```

7. Sarah takes the number 70 that she arrived at in step 5 and adds it to her resting heart rate of 72 (step 2) to arrive at her *minimum* training heart rate of 142. During a workout session, Sarah's heartbeats per minute should not fall below 142.

```
 70    Number arrived at in step 5
+72    Sarah's resting heart rate (step 2)
142    Sarah's minimum training heart rate
```

8. Sarah takes the number 93 that she arrived at in step 6 and adds it to her resting heart rate of 72 (step 2) to arrive at her *maximum* training heart rate of 165. During a workout session, Sarah's heartbeats per minute should not exceed 165.

```
 93    Number arrived at in step 6
+72    Sarah's resting heart rate (step 2)
165    Sarah's maximum training heart rate
```

9. Sarah has established her training heart-rate zone to be between 142 and 165.

At the high point of her aerobic session, Sarah will want to exercise hard enough to produce anywhere from 142 to 165 (her training heart-rate zone) heartbeats per minute. If this is, or becomes, too easy for her, the multiplier that determines the intensity level should be increased (as seen in step 5). If, on the other hand, this exercise work is too strenuous for Sarah, she should recalculate her training level with a smaller multiplier (as seen in step 6).

MONITORING YOUR HEART RATE DURING WORKOUTS

Heart rates should be monitored several times during an aerobic exercise session. Your pre-exercise heart rate should be taken before warming up. Your training-level heart rate (page 175) should be monitored at the high point of the session. Finally, a pulse should be taken after three minutes into the cool-down session; this is the *recovery heart rate.* Consistency in this area allows you to measure your self-improvement. You will recover your resting heart rate more quickly as your aerobic fitness improves.

IMPORTANCE OF FLUIDS

It is very important to drink liquids before, during, and after low-impact aerobic workouts. If you are breastfeeding, you have to be especially careful that you do not become dehydrated. Some signs of dehydration include increased pulse rate, nausea, pale dry skin or flushed red skin, hyperventilation, and fatigue. The added accumulation of fluids in your body and the extra heat generated due to the production of milk for your baby increases the amount that you sweat. This increases your need for adequate fluids.

Fitness experts recommend that you drink beyond your thirst when you are exercising. Try to work out in light clothing, and lower the intensity of your workout if it is humid.

IMPORTANCE OF PROPER BREATHING

Your breathing is very important during the entire aerobic segment of your workout. Proper breathing prevents you from overworking (thereby overtaxing) your body. An aerobic workout is intended to challenge the cardiovascular system by increasing the demand for oxygen in the larger muscles of the body, especially in the legs. Oxygen is supplied to your body by the work of your pumping heart and your circulatory system. Your breathing should be steady and patterned using your nose and mouth. Your breathing should not interfere with your exercise routine.

Never hold your breath! Always inhale through your nose on recovery, and exhale through your mouth on execution of the exercise (i.e. during sit-ups, inhale when you return to the floor and exhale when you lift). If you find yourself running out of breath, work out on a lower level for a while. This can be done by lowering your arms or by using less height when kicking your legs.

The following Tune-In Breath should be used throughout the exercise session whenever a re-establishment of concentration or alignment is needed.

Tune-In Breath

Benefits

- Helps re-establish concentration when exercising
- Helps you focus in on your breathing pattern and postural alignment

Cautions and Comments

- Maintain proper posture.
- Do not let your shoulders fall forward.
- On inhalation, lift your heels if desired.

Directions

1. Stand with your feet apart, knees bent, buttocks tucked under, and hands crossed in front of your chest (Figure 11.14).
2. As you inhale through your nose, stretch your arms out and around bringing them up over your head. Straighten your legs, but do not lock your knees.
3. As you exhale through your mouth, reverse and return to the starting position.
4. Repeat as needed.

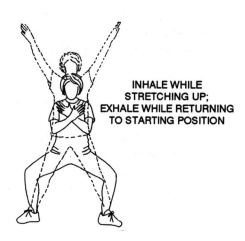

INHALE WHILE STRETCHING UP; EXHALE WHILE RETURNING TO STARTING POSITION

Figure 11.14 Tune-In Breath

DO'S AND DON'TS OF POSTPARTUM LOW-IMPACT AEROBICS*

- *Do* check with your health-care professional before initiating an aerobic program. This is very important if you desire to return to training within six weeks after delivery.
- *Do* give your body a chance to recover between aerobic workouts. Vary your routines so you do not practice aerobics two days in a row. On the alternate days do stretching or weight-training/Dyna-Band exercises (Chapter Twelve). If an occasional scheduling problem should occur, it is safe but not ideal to do aerobics for two consecutive days.

---

*These guidelines are according to Diane Milhan, PhD, PT, and Positive Parenting Fitness instructor.

- *Do* maintain proper body alignment while standing. During activity, constantly reassess your alignment. Softening your knees into bends will help prevent over-stretching; softening your pelvis into a slight pelvic tilt will help relieve backache caused by working with a hyperextended back.
- *Do* begin your workout with a warm-up period to raise your core body temperature.
- *Do* make a special effort to warm up any body area that remains sore from a previous workout.
- *Do* wear loose comfortable clothing and dress appropriately for the temperature of the room.
- *Do* try to set aside this time for yourself, free from all other distractions. If your baby is awake during this time, try to keep him entertained by placing him where he can see you move and can hear the music.
- *Do* support your breasts with a good sports bra (especially if you are breastfeeding).
- *Do* wear flexible shoes designed to accommodate the wide range of movements you will be going through. Some running shoes have wide soles that can cause stumbling when you move from side to side.
- *Do* drink liquids before, during, and after aerobic workouts.
- *Do* limit your joint movement to mid-range. In other words, do not swing to the very end of where your arms and legs can go. Hormones that were active during pregnancy to soften your ligaments remain active for some time after you've given birth. If you allow momentum or swing action to carry your limbs too far, you risk over-stretching and injury.
- *Do* repetitions of Kegels (page 104) if you experience leaking urine during a low-impact workout.

- *Don't* begin your aerobic workout without warming up. Legs, especially ankles, are prone to injury without a warm-up.
- *Don't* wear ankle weights when practicing low-impact aerobics. This added weight can cause severe bodily damage, especially in your lower back.
- *Don't* continue to work if you develop shortness of breath, especially extreme shortness of breath.
- *Don't* continue to work if you develop a cramp. Common places for muscle cramps are in the calf or hamstring (posterior thigh) muscles. You may also develop a "stitch" in the side of your trunk.
- *Don't* continue to work through unexplained or unusual symptoms.
- *Don't* exceed your projected training-level heart rate. If you have not figured your personal training level, do not allow your heart to exceed 140 beats per minute.
- *Don't* stop without performing cool-down exercises.
- *Don't* work in a poorly ventilated room.

- *Don't* hold your breath. You need oxygen, so continue to breathe normally. As the level of your work increases the faster your breathing will become until you reach a steady state. It is the maintenance of this steady state that produces the desired aerobic training effects (see page 173).
- *Don't* bounce individual body parts in an effort to stretch them. Slow, long stretches held in appropriate positions are the most effective.
- *Don't* use passive movements as part of your workout routine. All movements should be done actively using the strength of your muscles.
- *Don't* make a great effort to point your toes. This can result in calf muscle cramps. Take advantage of those steps that allow full placement of your feet on the floor and place your heels flat to counterbalance the toe pointing that is necessary.
- *Don't* use music that is too fast (over 160 beats per minute) or too slow (under 130 beats per minute).
- *Don't* continue to work if you are in any pain.
- *Don't* continue to repeatedly perform a movement that gives you a slipping or popping sensation. Even if pain-free, such movements should be stopped. Often, by shifting your position or by changing your range of motion, you can eliminate this popping sensation.

Low-Impact Aerobic-Workout Sequence

Benefits

- Promotes an increase in the efficiency of the heart, lungs, and cardiovascular system
- Strengthens the heart muscle so that an increased volume of blood is able to be pumped with each cardiac contraction
- Burns calories
- An aerobically fit individual can work longer, more vigorously, and can recover more quickly

Directions for Sample Low-Impact Routine

Keeping time to the beat of the music, perform the following movements. Always keep at least one foot on the floor and do not pause between movements. After completing the low-intensity phase, continue on to the high-intensity phase. Start out with 1 set of 8 movements for all steps (low and high-intensity phase) listed. Then gradually work to 5 sets for each step.

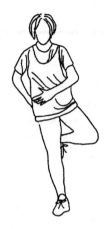

Figure 11.15 Sailor Step

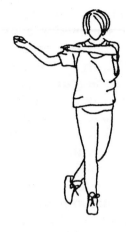

Figure 11.17 Arm Swing

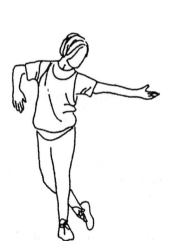

Figure 11.16 Side Reach

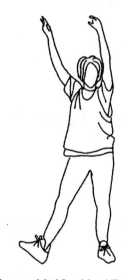

Figure 11.18 Heel Touch

1. *Sailor-Step*—Swing your arms in front and back while alternately lifting your heels (Figure 11.15).
2. *Side Reach*—Cross your left leg behind your right and touch your pointed toes to the ground. Simultaneously extend your right arm out to the side (Figure 11.16). Repeat from side to side.
3. *Arm Swing*—Cross your left leg behind your right and touch your pointed toes to the ground. Simultaneously swing both arms to the right (Figure 11.17). Repeat from side to side.
4. *Heel Touch*—Start out with hands at shoulder height. Extend hands to ceiling as you extend alternating heel touches on the floor (Figure 11.18).

Directions for Sample High-Intensity Phase

Add 8-32 counts of jogging in place or jumping jacks between all steps. Be creative and "free dance" or modify the sample movements presented.

1. *Lateral Elbow-to-Knee Touch*—With elbows elevated at shoulder height, lift your knees, one at a time, to your elbows (Figure 11.19). Keep arm movement at a minimum.

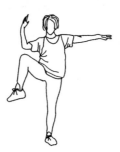

Figure 11.19   Lateral Elbow-to-Knee Touch

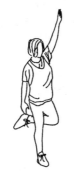

Figure 11.20   Rear-Heel Cross

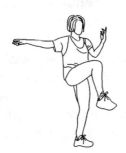

Figure 11.21   Front-Knee Touch

2. *Rear-Heel Cross*—Bend one of your legs behind you, touching your heel with your alternate hand, while raising your other arm into the air (Figure 11.20). Repeat on the other side.
3. *Front-Knee Touch*—Extend your arms out at shoulder height. Lift one knee, crossing your opposite elbow over to meet it (Figure 11.21). Repeat on the other side.

Cautions and Comments

- Individuals with specific needs, restrictions, or limitations (e.g. a known heart problem) should consult a physician before doing aerobic workouts.
- The best way to determine your training-level heart rate is by taking a physician-supervised stress test.
- Always begin your workout at a low-intensity level (arms and legs low) and gradually build up to higher-intensity movements (arms overhead, legs high).
- Never hold your breath! Breathe slowly and rhythmically. If necessary, perform Tune-In Breaths (page 179).
- To increase workout intensity, add wrist weights or lift your arms and legs higher during the movements. *Do not* use ankle weights for low-impact aerobics. These can cause shin splints or other injuries.
- If you add wrist weights, your arm movements should be controlled (not flaring about).
- Gradually add higher-intensity aerobic movements to your routine such as jogging or jumping jacks between steps.
- As your fitness level improves, increase the length of your high-impact aerobic interval.
- If you can't attend a Positive Parenting Fitness class in your town, you can work with some very fine low-impact aerobic video tapes (see page 301.)

Cool-Down Period

A proper cool-down period after a vigorous low-impact aerobic session is an essential part of a complete body workout. This transitional segment provides a gradual decrease in your heart rate until it is back to its normal state. It also prevents pooling of blood in the lower extremities. The suggestions listed below are simple, yet effective ways to cool down at the end of a workout. A period of 2-3 minutes is generally all the time that is necessary to properly cool down.

COOL-DOWN EXERCISE SUGGESTIONS

1. *Walking.* Simple low-intensity, low-impact movements when walking are quite effective.
2. *The Moon Salute* (page 159). This calming, cooling series is perfect as a cool-down exercise as well as for a warm-up.
3. *The Basic Eight* (page 136). Performing some or all of the postures found in this series is an excellent way to cool down.

Cautions and Comments

- Approximately 2-3 minutes after completion of an aerobic workout, you should see a decrease of 10 percent or more of your aerobic heart rate. Your recovery heart rate is a good indicator of your fitness level. The quicker the decrease in your heart rate after exercising, the higher your fitness level.
- If your heart rate remains elevated after two minutes of cool-down exercises, continue another minute or two until your heart rate is adequately lower.

REAPING THE REWARDS

Following "Your Complete Body Workout" may be quite a challenge for you at the start, but if you persevere you will notice an increase in energy as well as an all-around feeling of rejuvenation. Getting back into shape, both physically and mentally, is a slow-going process. Be proud for involving yourself in a workout program; you are doing something tangible to regain your shape and energy.

By this time, you may want to concentrate on those common "trouble spots" for most new moms: sagging tummies or large hips and thighs. Step #4 of the Positive Parenting Fitness program (coming up next in Chapter Twelve) concentrates on the fastest and safest exercises for dealing with these trouble spots. "Shaping Up and Strength Training for Motherhood Survival" includes creative exercises that you will enjoy practicing while working toward your goal: a shaped-up mom!

CHAPTER TWELVE
Step 4
Shaping Up and Strength Training for Motherhood Survival

Shaping up is the main goal of just about every new mother in my Positive Parenting Fitness classes. I suspect it is your goal as well. A toned, strengthened body will help you feel better and will make your mothering chores, such as carrying all of that baby equipment, easier. The fourth and final step of the Positive Parenting Fitness program is divided into two main categories: shaping up and strength training. The shaping-up section contains exercises that target those specific post-pregnancy trouble spots. They are designed to make you look and feel better. The strength-training category contains a set of imaginative, practical exercises geared toward helping you attain and maintain physical stamina.

You may be wondering how the exercises in this chapter differ from those in an aerobic workout. An aerobic workout is intended to challenge your cardiovascular system by increasing the demand for oxygen in the larger muscles of your body, especially those in the legs. Oxygen is supplied by the work of your pumping heart and your vascular system. The non-aerobic exercises found in this final step of the Positive Parenting Fitness program utilize a metabolic system of feeding those muscles that cannot be replenished by a flow of oxygen. Rather than having blood flowing constantly (as in an aerobic workout), non-aerobic exercise works your large muscles so specifically that the blood flow to them is reduced. Non-aerobic work produces fatigue in the muscles; the stress caused in the muscles by this fatigue is the mechanism of the training effect. It is during the resting phase between bouts of exercise that the muscles are rebuilding and increasing strength.

EXERCISE LEVELS

The shaping-up and strength-training exercises found in this chapter should be performed on the days you are resting between aerobic workouts (presented in Chapter Eleven). These exercises can be started approximately six weeks after a vaginal delivery and nine weeks after a Cesarean birth. Obviously, you will have to tune into your body and see when it is ready to begin these exercises.

The exercises in this chapter are presented by giving different levels of difficulty for each. Since your body is still healing after the birth of your child, always begin with the first-level directions.

Level-1 exercises use *imaginary resistance.* Here you work your muscles with effort *pretending* you are pushing against something. During your first few workout sessions, try to complete eight to twelve repetitions. When you have completed four sets of twelve repetitions, it is time to move on to the next level.

Level-2 exercises employ the use of wrist and ankle weights. These weights usually range from one-half to two pounds and provide more resistance than body weight alone. Weights used in strengthening exercises work your muscle fibers in order to shape and tone your body. They can be purchased in most sporting goods stores and fitness clubs.

Cautions When Working with Weights or Dyna-Bands

The exercises contained in this chapter are safe for most postpartum women. However, *stop immediately* and consult your physician if you experience any of the following symptoms:

- dizziness
- nausea
- heart palpitations
- severe and/or unusual pain

Women with the following conditions *should not* practice high-resistance exercises:

- hypertension
- a history of shoulder injuries or dislocations
- carpal tunnel syndrome
- any upper extremity disorder

In some cases, light-resistance exercises might be recommended but *only with the approval of your physician or physical therapist.*

Begin exercising with half-pound weights and gradually work your way up to a weight that does not limit your range of motion or reduce the number of comfortable repetitions you can do beyond eight. After two to three weeks of these exercises, you should be ready to move on to the next level.

Level-3 exercises, which use Dyna-Bands, are the most challenging. Dyna-Bands are thin sheets of latex that measure six inches wide by three feet long; they come with light, medium, or heavy resistance.

USING DYNA-BANDS

For use during Level-3 exercises, Dyna-Bands provide the most outside resistance for your muscles. As previously mentioned, these thin sheets of latex are made with light, medium, and heavy resistance.

When tying the Dyna-Band around your ankles, use a bow or knot. Tying a half-bow (Figure 12.1) is recommended because it can easily be untied. Leave one long end to grip with your hand. Figure 12.2 illustrates the two optional grips that can be used with your Dyna-Band. When exercising, try to maintain the Dyna-Band's natural width whenever possible; this will prevent it from sliding up your legs or digging into your hands.

You can protect your Dyna-Band by removing any rings before using it. Also, be careful if you have long, sharp fingernails for the Dyna-Band is easily ripped. Dyna-Bands should be stored out of direct sunlight and should be dusted with talcum powder at least once a week to help maintain their properties. Untie or flatten them out before storing. Dyna-Bands can be ordered through the *Be Healthy* catalog, page 315.

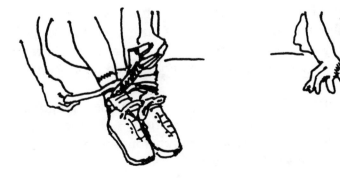

1. CAREFULLY WRAP DYNA-BAND AROUND ANKLES   2. TIE A HALF (SINGLE-LOOP) BOW

Figure 12.1 Tying the Dyna-Band

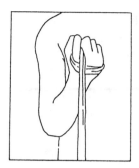

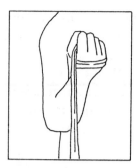

A. WRAP DYNA-BAND AROUND HAND ALLOWING IT
    TO RUN BETWEEN INDEX AND MIDDLE FINGER.
    KEEP WRIST STRAIGHT, PALM UP.

B. WRAP DYNA-BAND AROUND HAND ALLOWING IT
    TO RUN BETWEEN THUMB AND INDEX FINGER.
    KEEP WRIST STRAIGHT. CENTER FOREARM TO
    AVOID STRESS ON ELBOW.

Figure 12.2   Optional Grips for Dyna-Band

RULES AND TIPS FOR WEIGHT-TRAINING/DYNA-BAND WORKOUTS

- *Consult your physician or physical therapist before beginning any workout.*
- *Do not* use weights if you have high blood pressure or low blood sugar.
- If you have neck or lower-back problems, use extra caution. It is wise to see how your body reacts to this form of exercise, so take it slow.
- Wear comfortable clothing during exercise sessions.
- Drink an additional eight ounces of water daily to prevent dehydration during weight training.
- While exercising, do not hold your breath—breathe out through your mouth during exertion and inhale through your nose during release.
- Do not exceed two pounds of weight per arm when beginning your program. Start with half-pound weights and gradually build up.
- Light ankle weights should be used in controlled calisthenic exercises only. Be careful, ankle weights can cause painful shin splints or stress fractures when worn for non-control movements such as those in low-impact aerobics, running, or walking.
- Keep in mind that proper body alignment is essential for safety and proper results.
- Weights and Dyna-Bands should be used in slow, methodic, fluid movements. Avoid short, jerky motions.
- Quality, not quantity is important. These exercises develop muscle strength. Do not practice fast, jerky movements that rely solely on momentum.
- Aim to practice four sets of twelve repetitions comfortably before adding any additional weight or using a higher-resistance-level Dyna-Band.
- Use a modified range of motion during your exercises. Movement in the middle-range portion of a joint is the most taxing, yet the safest.
- Mellow pop, jazz, and modified disco (with no more than 120 beats per minute) work well with these exercises. Be creative with your music—let it suit your mood. Try ethnic, country, or modified-classical music occasionally.

Shaping-Up Workout

The following shaping-up exercises are designed to target those "trouble spots" that are concerning you. Exercises targeted at your waist, tummy, hips, thighs, and buttocks are all presented in this workout.

FOR THE FUTURE WAIST

Many of my students aren't sure if they will ever have a waistline again. I can almost guarantee that if you faithfully practice the following waist sequence, your waistline will return.

Waistline Twists

Benefits

- Strengthens and tones the waist
- Stretches and strengthens rectus and transverse abdominals and internal and external oblique muscle groups

Directions

1. Bend your knees and align them over your feet. *Do not move your hips.*
2. Hold your arms in the various positions shown in Figure 12.3.
3. Twist right and left with controlled motion, providing resistance for the working muscles.
4. Begin with 1 set of 8-12 repetitions for each position in Figure 12.3. In time, gradually increase the number of sets.

Cautions and Comments

- Do not twist forcefully.
- For the lateral reach, drop your shoulders directly to the side, not forward or backward.
- Use a broomstick for the twist with a stick.
- For maximum results, practice these waistline exercises in addition to Abdominal Curl-Ups (page 191).

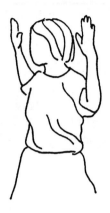

A. WITH UPRIGHT ARMS

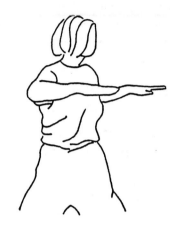

B. WITH LATERAL ARMS

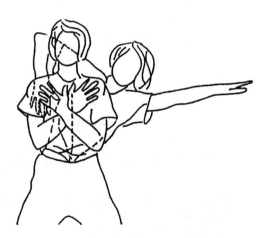

C. LATERAL REACH

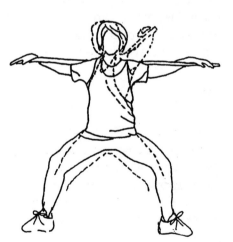

D. WITH A STICK

Figure 12.3   Waistline Twists

FOR THE SAGGING TUMMY

Your abdominal muscles will have been stretched to the limit by the end of your pregnancy, so it may take you quite a while to tone and strengthen them. The following progressive exercises will systematically strengthen and tone your abdominal muscles. Persevere and the desired results will come.

General Benefits for Abdominal Exercises

- Strengthens and tones abdominal muscles
- Strong abdominal muscles prevent postpartum backaches
- Strengthens and tones rectus and transverse abdominals and external and internal oblique muscles

Abdominal Curl-Ups

Directions

1. Contract your abdomen as you lift your shoulders and press your lower back firmly into the mat.
2. Keep your neck relaxed. In the variations where your head rests upon your hands, make sure you *do not pull your head up with your hands.*
3. Exhale when you lift up.
4. Begin with 1 set of 8-12 repetitions. In time, gradually increase the number of sets.
5. Begin with the Level-1 exercise variations until you are comfortable doing 4 sets of 8-12 repetitions. Then move on to the next level.
6. Follow the specific directions under Figures 12.4-12.10 for the variations.

Cautions and Comments

- If your neck is uncomfortable when you extend your arms in any of the variations, put your hand behind your head for support.
- Your goal should be to work up to as many repetitions as you can.

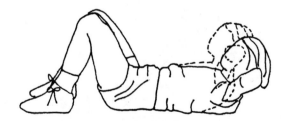

HEELS FLAT, HANDS BEHIND HEAD

Figure 12.4 Level-1 Abdominal Curl-Ups: Variation I

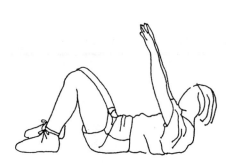

ARMS EXTENDED UP IN THE AIR

Figure 12.5   Level-1 Abdominal Curl-Ups:
Variation II

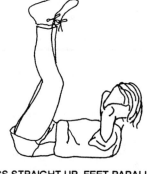

LEGS STRAIGHT UP, FEET PARALLEL

Figure 12.8   Level-3 Abdominal Curl-Ups:
Variation I

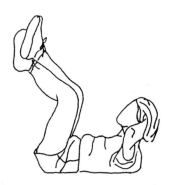

ANKLES CROSSED, KNEES FLEXED

Figure 12.6   Level-2 Abdominal Curl-Ups:
Variation I

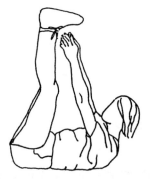

ARMS AND LEGS EXTENDED IN AIR

Figure 12.9   Level-3 Abdominal Curl-Ups:
Variation II

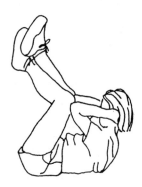

MAKING CONTACT WITH ELBOWS AND KNEES

Figure 12.7   Level-2 Abdominal Curl-Ups:
Variation II

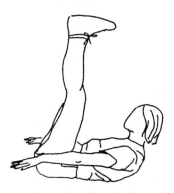

ARMS PARALLEL TO FLOOR

Figure 12.10   Level-3 Abdominal Curl-Ups:
Variation III

Abdominal Twists

Directions

1. Lie on your back with your knees bent and one leg crossed.
2. Put your hands behind your head, curl forward, and twist bringing your right elbow to your left knee (Figure 12.11).
3. Complete 1 set of 8-12 repetitions, then repeat on the other side. In time, gradually increase the number of sets.
4. Follow the specific directions under Figures 12.12-12.13.

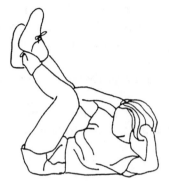

KNEES BENT, ANKLES CROSSED

Figure 12.12 Level-2 Abdominal Twist

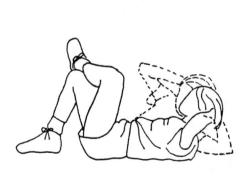

Figure 12.11 Level-1 Abdominal Twist

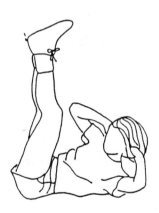

LEGS STRAIGHT UP, FEET PARALLEL

Figure 12.13 Level-3 Abdominal Twist

Lower-Abdominal Curl-Ups

Directions

1. Lie on your back with the soles of your feet together. Bend your knees and drop them to the sides forming a diamond shape.
2. Put your hands behind your head and curl up.
3. Begin with 8-12 repetitions. In time, gradually increase the number of sets.

4. Follow the specific directions under Figures 12.14 and 12.15 for the variations. Directions are for all levels.

Cautions and Comments

- Do not arch your back.
- Do not hold your breath. Exhale each time you curl up.

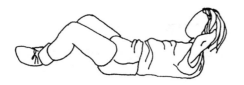

HANDS BEHIND HEAD

Figure 12.14   Lower-Abdominal Curl-Up: Variation I

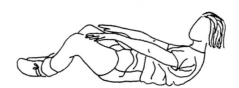

ARMS EXTENDED

Figure 12.15   Lower-Abdominal Curl-Up: Variation II

TO REDUCE HIPS, THIGHS, AND BUTTOCKS

Leg Extensions

Benefits

- Tones and trims the upper thighs
- Strengthens and tones the quadricep muscles; rectus femoris; vastus lateralis, medialis, and intermedius

Directions for Level 1 and Level 2

1. Lie on your back with your knees bent and aligned with your hips.
2. Place your hands under your lower back and keep your lower legs parallel to the floor.
3. Using imaginary resistance, *slowly* extend one leg at a time toward the ceiling (Figure 12.16). *Do not lock your knees.* Slowly return to the starting position. Repeat with the other leg.
4. Begin at Level 1 until you are comfortable doing 4 sets of 8-12 repetitions with each leg. Then move on to the next level.
5. Add ankle weights for Level 2 and follow the same directions as above (Figure 12.17).

Directions for Level 3

1. Sit, leaning back with your elbows bent, knees bent, and feet on the floor. Your back should be curled slightly inward.
2. With a Dyna-Band loosely tied around your ankles, extend one leg at a time keeping both knees aligned (Figure 12.18).
3. Begin with 1 set of 8-12 repetitions for each leg. Gradually increase the number of sets.

Cautions and Comments

- Do not hold your breath. Exhale on each exertion.
- Proper body positioning will make this exercise easier to do.

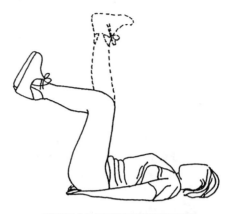

USING IMAGINARY RESISTANCE

Figure 12.16   Level-1 Leg Extension

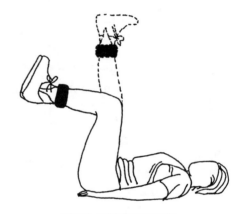

USING ANKLE WEIGHTS

Figure 12.17   Level-2 Leg Extension

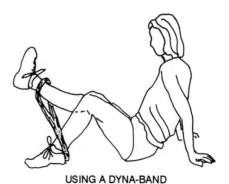

USING A DYNA-BAND

Figure 12.18   Level-3 Leg Extension

Leg Curls

Benefits

- Shapes up the muscles at the back of the thighs
- Strengthens and tones the hamstring muscle group: biceps femoris, semitendinosus, and semimembranosus

Directions for Level 1 and Level 2

1. Position yourself on your knees and elbows. Extend one leg back so that it aligns with your torso.
2. Keep your abdominals pulled in and *do not arch your back.*
3. Slowly bend your knee and pull your heel in toward your buttocks (Figure 12.19).
4. Begin with 1 set of 8-12 repetitions, then repeat with the other leg.
5. When you are comfortable doing 4 sets of 8-12 repetitions with each leg, move on to Level 2.

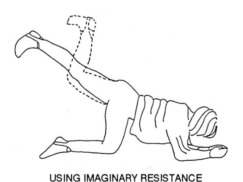

USING IMAGINARY RESISTANCE

Figure 12.19   Level-1 Leg Curls

6. Add ankle weights for Level 2 and follow the same directions as above (Figure 12.20).

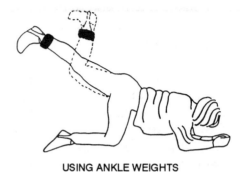

USING ANKLE WEIGHTS

Figure 12.20   Level-2 Leg Curls

Directions for Level 3

1. Make a one-looped bow with your Dyna-Band (page 187) and tie it around your ankles.
2. Lie on your stomach and keep your legs flat on the mat while you slowly bend one of your knees, pulling your heel toward your buttocks (Figure 12.21). *Do not arch your back.*
3. Begin with 1 set of 8-12 repetitions for each leg. Gradually increase sets.

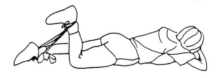

USING A DYNA-BAND

Figure 12.21   Level-3 Leg Curls

Cautions and Comments

- If you feel a strain on your lower back, bring your working leg to a lower level.
- Do not hold your breath.

Outer-Thigh Slimmers

Benefits

- Strengthens and tones the outer thighs and buttocks
- Strengthens tensor fasciae latae; gluteus maximus, medius, and minimus

Directions for Level 1 and Level 2

1. Lie on your side and support your torso by leaning on your elbow. Bring your knees forward in a 90° angle to your hip.
2. Without shifting your upper body, slowly lift your top leg and extend it while keeping your bottom knee at a 90° angle.
3. Raise your extended leg up, then lower it (Figure 12.22).
4. Do 1 set of 8-12 repetitions, then repeat with the other leg.
5. When you are comfortable doing 4 sets of 8-12 repetitions on each side, move on to Level 2.
6. Add ankle weights for Level 2 and follow the same directions as above.
7. Follow the specific directions under Figures 12.23 and 12.24 for variations.

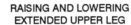
RAISING AND LOWERING EXTENDED UPPER LEG

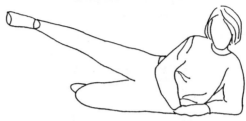

Figure 12.22   Levels -1 and 2 Outer-Thigh Slimmers: Variation I
(Use ankle weight on working leg for Level 2)

RAISING AND LOWERING BENT LEG

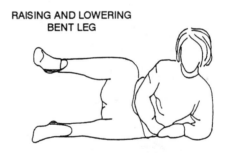

Figure 12.23   Levels -1 and 2 Outer-Thigh Slimmers: Variation II
(Use ankle weight on working leg for Level 2)

RAISING AND LOWERING UPPER LEG THAT IS EXTENDED FORWARD

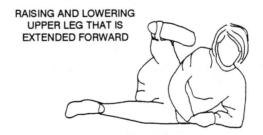

Figure 12.24   Levels-1 and 2 Outer-Thigh Slimmers: Variation III
(Use ankle weight on working leg for Level 2)

Directions for Level 3

1. Lie flat on your stomach with a Dyna-Band tied around your ankles.
2. Leading with your heels, pull your legs apart and slowly let your toes slide along the mat until they are back in the starting position (Figure 12.25). This Level-3 exercise can also be done while lying on your side (Figure 12.26).

3. Begin with 1 set of 8-12 repetitions. Gradually increase the number of sets.

Cautions and Comments

- Be sure you are in the proper position before beginning.
- Do not hold your breath. Exhale on each exertion.

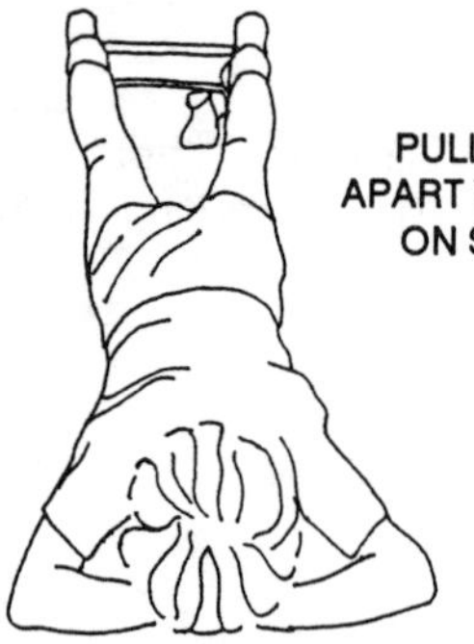

PULLING LEGS
APART WHILE LYING
ON STOMACH

PULLING LEGS APART
WHILE LYING ON SIDE

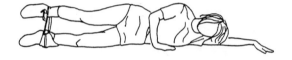

Figure 12.25   Level-3 Outer-Thigh
Slimmer: Variation I
(Dyna-Band around ankles)

Figure 12.26   Level-3 Outer-Thigh
Slimmers: Variation II
(Dyna-Band around ankles)

Inner-Thigh Slimmers

Benefits

- Strengthens and tones the inner thighs
- Stretches and strengthens pectineus, adductor longus and magnus, and gracilis muscles

Directions for Level 1 and Level 2

Variation I:
1. Lie on your side and support your torso by leaning on your elbow.
2. Bend your upper knee and place your foot flat on the mat behind your working (lower) leg.
3. Your working leg should be extended with knee bent slightly and foot facing forward.
4. Leading with your heel, lift your working leg (Figure 12.27).
5. Begin with 1 set of 8-12 repetitions, then repeat with the other leg.
6. When you are comfortable doing 4 sets of 8-12 repetitions with each leg, move on to Level 2.
7. Add an ankle weight to your working leg for Level 2. Follow the same directions as above.

Variation II:

1. Lie on your back with your hands, palms down, under your buttocks.
2. Raise both legs into the air and place the soles of your feet together.
3. Bend your knees and drop them out to the sides, forming a diamond shape (Figure 12.28).
4. Slowly straighten your legs back up into the air, bringing your knees together.
5. Begin with 1 set of 8-12 repetitions.
6. When you are comfortable doing 4 sets of 8-12 repetitions, move on to Level 2.
7. Add ankle weights for Level 2 and follow the same directions as above.

Directions for Level 3

1. Tie a Dyna-Band around your ankles and stand with your feet together.
2. Rotate one leg outward and extend it forward, pushing with your heel (Figure 12.29).
3. Slowly return your foot to the starting position.
4. Begin with 1 set of 8-12 repetitions, then repeat with the other leg. Gradually increase the number of sets.

Cautions and Comments

- Before starting the Level-3 exercise, make sure your hips are tucked under and that you are in a proper standing position (page 116).
- Do not hold your breath. Exhale on each exertion.

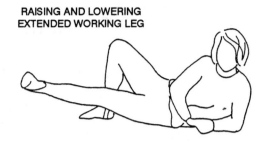

RAISING AND LOWERING EXTENDED WORKING LEG

Figure 12.27 Levels-1 and 2 Inner-Thigh Slimmers: Variation I
(Use ankle weight for Level 2)

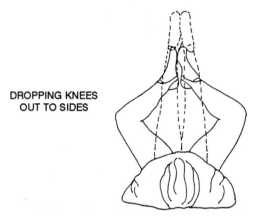

DROPPING KNEES OUT TO SIDES

Figure 12.28 Levels-1 and 2 Inner-Thigh Slimmers: Variation II
(Use ankle weight for Level 2)

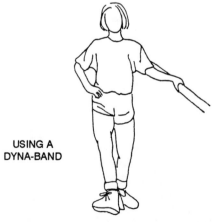

USING A DYNA-BAND

Figure 12.29 Level-3 Inner-Thigh Slimmer

Standing Hip Flexor

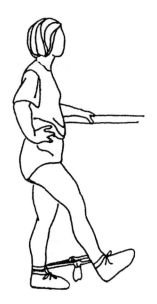

Figure 12.30   Standing Hip Flexor

Benefits

- Slims hips and upper thighs
- Strengthens and tones iliopsoas muscle group and upper-thigh muscles (above quadriceps)

Directions

1. For this Level-3 exercise, tie a Dyna-Band around your ankles and stand with your feet together and knees slightly bent.
2. Extend one leg as far forward as possible without leaning forward (Figure 12.30).
3. Slowly return foot to starting position.
4. Begin with 1 set of 8-12 repetitions, then repeat with the other leg. Gradually increase the number of sets.

Cautions and Comments

- Make sure you maintain good postural alignment.
- Set a goal of 4 sets of 12 repetitions.

Buttocks Slimmer

Benefits

- Shapes and tones the buttocks
- Strengthens and tones gluteus maximus, medius, and minimus; and the hamstring muscles

Directions

1. For this Level 3 exercise, tie a Dyna-Band around your ankles and stand with your feet together, knees slightly bent.
2. Extend one leg back as far as you can (Figure 12.31). Make sure your front foot is flat and you lead with the heel of your back foot. Lean slightly forward on the exertion to maintain spinal align
3. Slowly return foot to starting position.
4. Begin with 1 set of 8-12 repetitions, then repeat with the other leg. Gradually increase the number of sets.

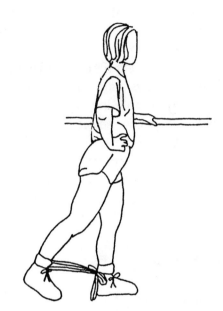

Figure 12.32 Buttocks Slimmer

Cautions and Comments

- Make sure you maintain good postural alignment.
- Set a goal of 4 sets of 12 repetitions.

Strength-Training Workout

Aren't you surprised that your baby and all of that baby equipment are so heavy? The following weight-training and Dyna-Band exercises are the perfect answer for shaping up and developing strength for your new mothering role. These exercises are designed to help you maintain muscle tissue while preventing loss of bone mass and osteoporosis. They will also help strengthen your muscles, thereby preventing postural and lower-back problems.

Most of the exercises found in this strength-training workout can be practiced on three levels. Always start on Level 1 by practicing the exercises with imaginary resistance. Begin by completing one set of eight to twelve repetitions for each exercise during the first few practice sessions. Gradually begin to add additional sets of repetitions. When you have completed four sets of twelve repetitions comfortably in Level 1, you can move on to Level 2 by completing the same exercises with wrist or ankle weights. When you comfortably complete four sets of twelve repetitions with weights, it is time to move on to Level 3 by adding a Dyna-Band while doing the exercises. A Dyna-Band will provide the greatest resistance.

CHEST EXERCISES

General Benefits

- •Strengthens and tones the arm and chest area
- •Stretches and strengthens pectoralis major and anterior deltoid muscles

Chest Presses

Directions

1. Hold your arms laterally with your elbows bent at 90° angles. Inhale.
2. Slowly exhale as you squeeze your elbows together in front of you (Figure 12.32).
3. Begin by doing 1 set of 12 repetitions.
4. When you can comfortably do 4 sets of 12 repetitions, move to Level 2 by adding wrist weights (Figure 12.33).
5. When you can comfortably do 4 sets of 12 repetitions with wrist weights, move to Level 3 by doing this exercise with a Dyna-Band. Hold one end of the Dyna-Band in each hand; it should go behind your back and under each arm (Figure 12.34).

Cautions and Comments

• Chest presses work many sets of muscles in your chest and back in ways that they are not used to. You may find surprising resistance to these movements in the beginning.
• Chest presses help strengthen and tone your upper body.

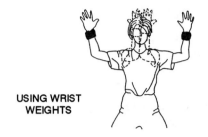

USING WRIST WEIGHTS

Figure 12.33 Level-2 Chest Press
(inhale in open position, exhale on squeeze)

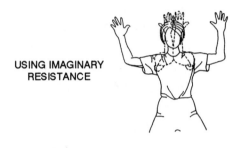

USING IMAGINARY RESISTANCE

Figure 12.32 Level-1 Chest Press
(inhale in open position, exhale on squeeze)

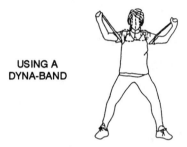

USING A DYNA-BAND

Figure 12.34 Level-3 Chest Press
(inhale in open position, exhale on squeeze)

Modified Push-Ups

Directions (Level 1 only)

1. Get on hands and knees in push-up position. Cross ankles (Figure 12.35).
2. Inhale and lower yourself to mat.
3. Exhale and return to start position.
4. Start with 1 set of 12 repetitions.

Cautions and Comments

• Make sure your back is flat.
• Movement should occur at the elbow and shoulder joints.
• If this version is too difficult you can practice a wall push-up instead.

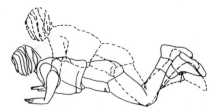

Figure 12.35 Modified Push-Ups
(inhale and lower, exhale on return)

BACK EXERCISES

General Benefits

- Eliminates backaches
- Strengthens and tones upper, middle, and lower back
- Stretches and strengthens the scalenus, deltoid, and rotator cuff muscle groups

Horizontal Arm Pull

Directions

1. Inhale. Extend your arms in front so they are parallel to the floor.
2. Exhale as you slowly pull your elbows back and squeeze your shoulder blades together (Figure 12.36).
3. Begin by doing 1 set of 12 repetitions.
4. When you can comfortably do 4 sets of 12 repetitions, move to Level 2 by adding wrist weights (Figure 12.37).
5. When you can do 4 sets of 12 repetitions with wrist weights, move on to Level 3 by doing this exercise with a Dyna-Band wrapped around your wrists (Figure 12.38).

Cautions and Comments

- Remember to breathe correctly.
- Keep your arms parallel to the floor.

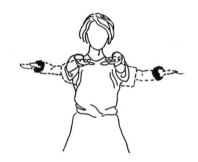

USING WRIST WEIGHTS

Figure 12.37 Level-2 Horizontal Arm Pulls
(inhale in starting position, exhale on squeeze)

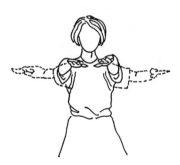

USING IMAGINARY RESISTANCE

Figure 12.36 Level-1 Horizontal Arm Pulls
(inhale in starting position, exhale on squeeze)

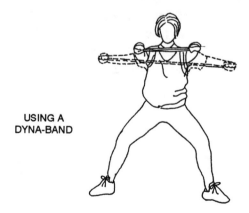

USING A
DYNA-BAND

Figure 12.38 Level-3 Horizontal Arm Pulls
(inhale in starting position, exhale on squeeze)

Back Toner

Directions

1. Inhale through your nose as you extend your arms over your head.
2. Exhale through your mouth as you bend your elbows and bring your arms to your sides pulling your elbows toward your body (Figure 12.39). This movement should be done slowly and with control.
3. Begin by doing 1 set of 12 repetitions.
4. When you can comfortably do 4 sets of 12 repetitions, move to Level 2 by adding wrist weights (Figure 12.40).
5. When you can comfortably do 4 sets of 12 repetitions with wrist weights, move on to Level 3 by doing this exercise with a Dyna-Band. Hold one end of the Dyna-Band in each hand; when pulling your elbows toward your body (step 2), bring the Dyna-Band back behind your head (Figure 12.41).

Cautions and Comments

- Remember to breathe correctly. Exhale through your mouth on exertion; inhale through your nose on release.
- Keep the movements controlled (don't rush through them).

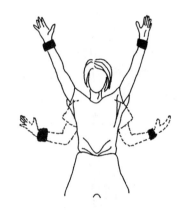

USING WRIST WEIGHTS

Figure 12.40 Level-2 Back Toner
(inhale when extending arms up, exhale when bringing arms down)

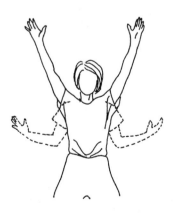

USING IMAGINARY RESISTANCE

Figure 12.39 Level-1 Back Toner
(inhale when extending arms up, exhale when bringing arms down)

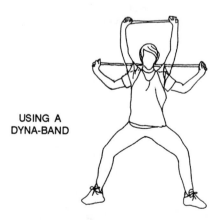

USING A DYNA-BAND

Figure 12.41 Level-3 Back Toner
(inhale when extending arms up, exhale when bringing arms down)

Lower-Back Strengthener

Directions (Level 3 only)

1. Grip or wrap the ends of a Dyna-Band in each hand.
2. With your knees bent, lean forward at the waist and place the center of the Dyna-Band securely under your feet. Inhale.
3. Exhale through your mouth as you slowly raise up to a standing position (Figure 12.42).
4. Return to starting position.
5. Begin by doing 1 set of 12 repetitions. Gradually increase the amount of repetitions. Your goal should be to complete 4 sets of 12 repetitions.

Cautions and Comments

- Do not arch your back or lean backward while in the standing position.
- Through strengthening the lower-back muscles, this exercise helps protect and stabilize your spine.
- Do not perform if you have a history of back problems.

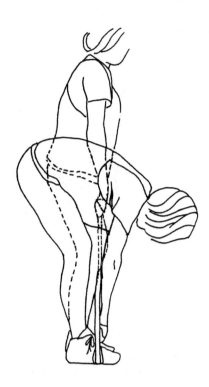

SECURING CENTER OF DYNA-BAND UNDER FEET

Figure 12.42 Lower-Back Strengthener (inhale in start position, exhale when raising up)

SHOULDER AND ARM EXERCISES

Lateral Arm Raises

Benefits

- Strengthens shoulder muscles
- Stretches and strengthens the deltoid muscles

Directions

1. Stand with your elbows in a bent position at your sides with your forearms parallel to the floor. Inhale.
2. Keeping your elbows bent, slowly exhale and raise your arms until your elbows are parallel with your shoulders (Figure 12.43).
3. Slowly return to the starting position.
4. Begin by doing 1 set of 12 repetitions.
5. When you can comfortably complete 4 sets of 12 repetitions, move to Level 2 by adding wrist weights (Figure 12.44).
6. When you can comfortably complete 4 sets of 12 repetitions with wrist weights, move to Level 3 by doing this exercise with a Dyna-Band. Wrap one end of the Dyna-Band around your hand and place the other end securely under your foot. Exhale as you bend your elbow and raise your arm until it is parallel with your shoulder (Figure 12.45).

Cautions and Comments

- Move your arms only, not your entire body.
- Be aware of your posture.

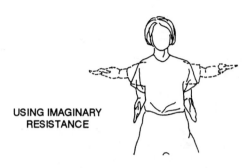

USING IMAGINARY RESISTANCE

Figure 12.43 Level-1 Lateral Arm Raises
(inhale in start position, exhale when raising arms)

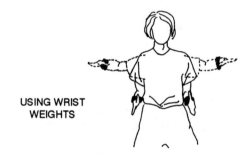

USING WRIST WEIGHTS

Figure 12.44 Level-2 Lateral Arm Raises
(inhale in start position, exhale when raising arms)

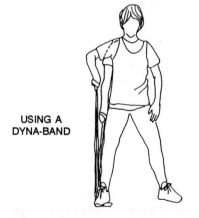

USING A DYNA-BAND

Figure 12.45 Level-3 Lateral Arm Raises
(inhale in start position, exhale when raising arm)

Arm Curls

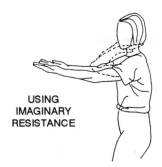

USING
IMAGINARY
RESISTANCE

Figure 12.46 Level-1 Arm Curls
(inhale with extended arms, exhale while bringing
hands to shoulders)

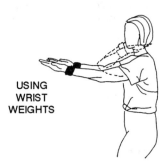

USING
WRIST
WEIGHTS

Figure 12.47 Level-2 Arm Curls
(inhale with extended arms, exhale while bringing
hands to shoulders)

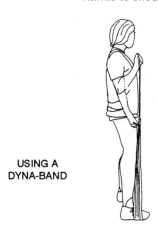

USING A
DYNA-BAND

Figure 12.48 Level-3 Arm Curls
(inhale with extended arms, exhale while bringing
hands to shoulders)

Benefits

• Strengthens and tones upper arms
• Helps prevent "jiggly" arms
• Stretches and strengthens biceps bra-
chii muscles

Directions

1. Stand or sit with your arms extended forward (elbows slightly bent) and parallel to the floor. Inhale.
2. With palms facing upward, slowly bring your hands up toward your shoulders while exhaling through your mouth (Figure 12.46).
3. Return to starting position.
4. Begin by doing 1 set of 12 repetitions.
5. When you can comfortably do 4 sets of 12 repetitions, move to Level 2 by adding wrist weights (Figure 12.47).
6. When you can comfortably do 4 sets of 12 repetitions with wrist weights, move to Level 3 by doing this exercise with a Dyna-Band. While stepping securely on the middle of the Dyna-Band, hold one end in each hand. Exhale as you slowly bring your hands up to your shoulders (Figure 12.48).

Cautions and Comments

• Make sure your arms are doing all the work.
• Be aware of your posture.
• Remember to breathe properly.

Upper-Arm Toners

Benefits

- Strengthens the muscles located in the back of the upper arms
- Stretches and strengthens the triceps and brachii muscles

Directions

1. Leaning forward slightly, raise your arms laterally with your elbows bent and parallel to the floor. Inhale.
2. Slowly press your hands out to the sides, extending your arms (Figure 12.49). Exhale. (Do not lock elbows.)
3. Return to the starting position.
4. Begin by doing 1 set of 12 repetitions.
5. When you can comfortably do 4 sets of 12 repetitions, move to Level 2 by adding wrist weights (Figure 12.50).
6. When you can comfortably do 4 sets of 12 repetitions with wrist weights, move to Level 3 by doing this exercise with a Dyna-Band wrapped around each hand (Figure 12.51).

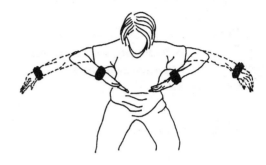

USING WRIST WEIGHTS

Figure 12.50 Level-2 Upper-Arm Toners
(inhale in starting position, exhale on extension)

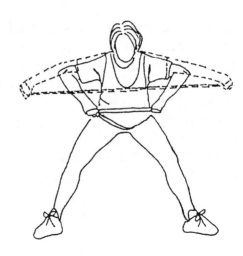

USING A DYNA-BAND

Figure 12.51 Level-3 Upper-Arm Toners:
Variation I
(inhale in starting position, exhale on extension)

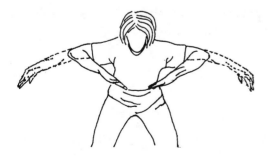

USING IMAGINARY RESISTANCE

Figure 12.49 Level-1 Upper-Arm Toners
(inhale in starting position, exhale on extension)

Directions for Level 3: Variation II

1. Hold one end of the Dyna-Band comfortably behind your neck and the other end behind your lower back (Figure 12.52). Inhale.
2. Slowly extend the top of your arm up while keeping the elbow close to your ear. Exhale.
3. Repeat 12 times with each arm.
4. Begin by completing 1 set of 12 repetitions, then gradually increase the number of sets.

Cautions and Comments

•Be aware of your posture.
•Make sure you breathe properly.

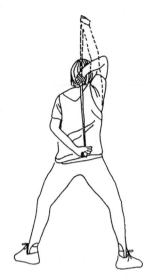

USING A DYNA-BAND

Figure 12.52   Level-3 Upper-Arm Toners:
Variation II
(inhale in starting position, exhale on extension)

END-OF-SESSION STRETCHES

It is helpful to end your workout session with some stretches. Through stretching, any lactic acid that is produced during your workout will be washed off, preventing aches and pains tomorrow. End-of-session stretches should be relaxing, refreshing, and enjoyable. They should make you feel good. Because your flexibility is improved at this time, your risk of injury is very low.

Approximately 7-10 minutes of stretching at the end of the workout is all that is needed. You can choose any of the warm-up stretches or static stretches found in Chapter Eleven. The Basic Eight or the Sun and Moon Salutes (Chapter Ten) are also excellent for end-of-session stretches.

PART III

A Family Affair

CHAPTER THIRTEEN
Family Exercise Routines

The family exercise routines have been divided into three main sections. The first section provides exercises specifically for moms and babies. The second section includes exercises designed for babies and dads, while the final section includes exercises that involve the entire family.

These simple, comprehensive, fun-to-do exercises will not only help keep you in shape but will help strengthen those all-important family ties.

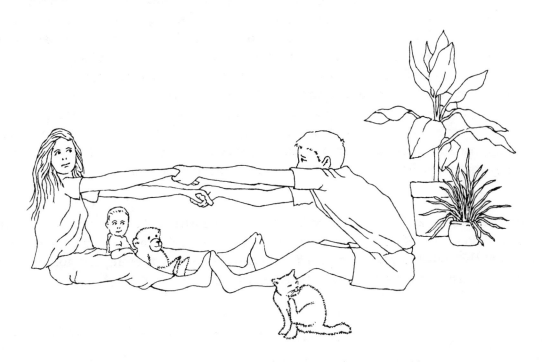

Exercise Routines for Mommy and Baby

Exercising with your baby can be fun and very energizing. The exercises found in this section are designed to be fun and entertaining for both you and your baby, while providing you with a comprehensive workout.* The entire routine takes only twenty to thirty minutes, which can be easily included in your daily schedule. Familiarize yourself with all of the exercises. Try them with a doll before practicing them with your baby.

PRACTICE GUIDELINES

1. **Start slowly and minimize the movements.** Very young babies can be easily startled or overstimulated. You probably won't get through the entire workout the first few times. During each session try to introduce at least one new exercise.
2. **Use your creativity!** You can put your whole routine to music. The *Morning Magic* tape (page 312) has a wonderful selection of children's songs appropriate for these exercises. Incorporating toys or wearing colorful hair ribbons can enhance your baby's enjoyment and, therefore, extend your workout time.
3. **Change your baby's position.** If there is an exercise that your baby finds uncomfortable or is adverse to, try holding him in a different way. Some babies like to be cradled while others insist on being held in a sitting position. A simple adjustment may be all that's needed. Otherwise, you may have to eliminate that exercise for a while, but be sure to try it again in a few weeks. It may end up being one of your baby's favorites.
4. **Concentrate on form.** Although the emphasis here is on fun, it's important that you don't sacrifice correct posture and form. *Never let your back arch while lifting your baby during these exercises or during any of your other daily activities.* When lifting, always remember to pull in your tummy before you pick up the baby. This will give your back support and prevent straining. You might also try doing a small *pelvic tilt* (lifting your pubic bone and tucking your seat under) while you lift.

   Follow these guidelines and the following exercise instructions carefully. These exercises will flow naturally, one into the other, if practiced in the sequence given. You will find that through this playful interaction, you will be strengthening and toning your body, while strengthening the bond between you and your baby.

---

*Liz Schneider, Positive Parenting Fitness Instructor, New York City, created the exercises found in this section. See page 313 for her video.

Good-Morning Stretch

Benefits

- Warms up the legs, back, and arms
- Stretches the gastrocnemius muscle group; hamstrings, lumbar erector spinae, gluteals, latissimus dorsi, and anterior neck muscles

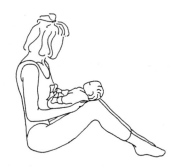

A. STARTING POSITION

Directions

1. Begin in a sitting position with your knees together and slightly bent. Your feet should be flat on the floor.
2. Lay the baby on your lap with his back against your thighs and his feet against your chest (Figure 13.1A). Hold him under his armpits.
3. Straighten your legs as you slide the baby down your legs towards your ankles, stretching as far as you can (Figure 13.1B).
4. Lift the baby up over your head (Figure 13.1C).
5. Return to starting position.
6. Repeat 4-8 times.

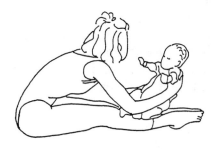

B. STRETCHING FORWARD

Cautions and Comments

- Keep your arms slightly bent when lifting.
- Make sure you pull in your abdominal muscles before lifting.
- Breathe deeply to increase the oxygen flow to your muscles and to begin warming up your body.

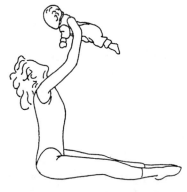

C. LIFTING THE BABY

Figure 13.1 Good-Morning Stretch

Fanny Walks

Benefits

- Warms up the hips and thighs
- Strengthens the quadratus lumborum, obliques, hamstrings, gluteals, thoracic and lumbar erector spinae

Directions

1. Begin in a sitting position with your back erect and your legs straight out.
2. Lay the baby on your lap facing you. Support his back with one hand and cup his head with your other hand (Figure 13.2).
3. Move your right hip and leg forward, then your left hip and leg.
4. Alternate right and left 8 times forward, then 8 times back.

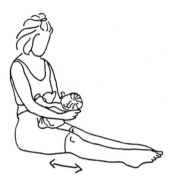

Figure 13.2 Fanny Walks

Cautions and Comments

- Keep your back straight and tummy tucked in.
- Have fun with this one — babies love it!

Curl-Backs with Baby

Benefits

- Warms lower back area
- Strengthens iliopsoas muscle group and rectus and oblique abdominals

Directions

1. Sit with your knees slightly bent.
2. Lay the baby on your lap with his back against your thighs and his feet against your chest (Figure 13.3A). Hold his hands (he can grip your thumbs).
3. Round your back and exhale while bringing your lower back close to the floor (Figure 13.3B).
4. Inhale and return to the start position.
5. Repeat 8 times.

Cautions and Comments

- Do not go back so far as to touch your waist to the floor.
- Flex your feet as you curl back if this is more comfortable for you.
- Don't let your tummy bulge as you curl back. Envision yourself pulling your belly button in toward the spine.
- Move slowly in a flowing motion.

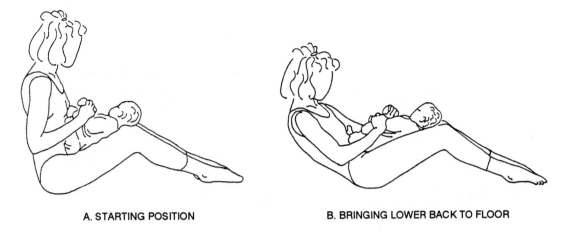

A. STARTING POSITION   B. BRINGING LOWER BACK TO FLOOR

Figure 13.3   Curl-Backs with Baby

Airplane Ride

Benefits

- Stretches and releases tension in the lower back
- Relaxes the entire back

Directions

1. Begin by lying on your back with your knees bent and pulled close to your chest.
2. Rest your baby's tummy on your shins and hold out his arms like airplane wings (Figure 13.4).
3. Rock gently from side to side, stopping your movement on each side with your elbow.
4. Repeat 4-8 times.

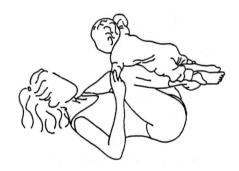

Figure 13.4   Airplane Ride

Cautions and Comments

- With a very tiny baby, you may have to hold the baby's torso and save the airplane wings for later.
- Make sure to rock slowly and gently.

Kiss-the-Baby Sit-Ups

Benefits

- Strengthens all abdominal muscles
- Strengthens anterior cervical muscles (sternocleidomastoid), obliques, rectus abdominalis
- Stretches cervical, thoracic, and lumbar erector spinae; gluteals

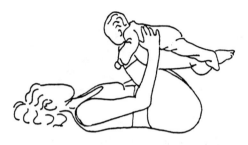

A. STARTING POSITION

Directions

1. Lie on your back with knees bent and pulled close to your chest.
2. Rest the baby's tummy on your shins (Figure 13.5A).
3. Curl your head and shoulders up off the floor and exhale while reaching up to kiss your baby (Figure 13.5B).
4. Inhale while lowering back to the starting position.
5. Repeat 5-10 times.

Cautions and Comments

- Make sure you bring your upper body up to reach the baby. Don't cheat by bringing your knees down.
- Start out by doing a few, then add one more sit-up every other time you work out.

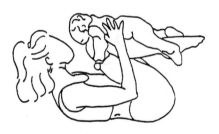

B. REACHING UP TO KISS BABY

Figure 13.5 Kiss-the-Baby Sit-Ups

Baby Back-and-Forth

Benefits

- Strengthens the lower abdominal muscles
- Strengthens obliques and transversus abdominalis and quadriceps
- Stretches lumbar erector spinae, gluteals

Directions

1. Lie on your back with your knees bent and pulled close to your chest.
2. Rest your baby's tummy on your shins while holding him by the arms and shoulders (Figure 13.6A).
3. Reach out with your toes until your knees are directly over your hips (Figure 13.6B).
4. Bring your knees back close to your chest.
5. Repeat back and forth 8 times.

Cautions and Comments

- Always keep your shins parallel to the floor for proper alignment.
- Keep your lower back pressed tightly against the floor.
- Your head and shoulders can rest on the floor or curl up slightly.

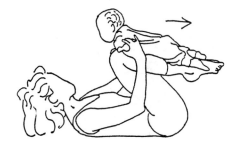

A. STARTING POSITION

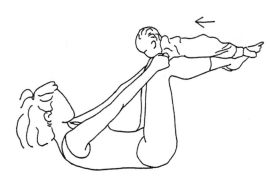

B. REACHING OUT WITH YOUR TOES

Figure 13.6 Baby Back-and-Forth

Full Curl-Ups with Baby

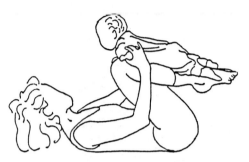

A. STARTING POSITION

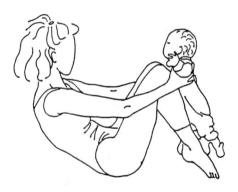

B. CURLING UP

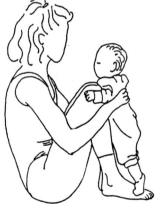

C. COMPLETED CURL-UP

Figure 13.7 Full Curl-Ups

Benefits

- Strengthens front abdominal muscles
- Strengthens rectus and oblique abdominals and the iliopsoas muscle group
- Stretches thoracic and lumbar erector spinae

Directions

1. Lie on your back with your knees bent and pulled close to your chest.
2. Lay your baby's tummy on your shins and hold him under his armpits (Figure 13.7A).
3. Curl all the way up to a sitting position (Figures 13.7B and 13.7C).
4. Lower yourself back to the starting position.
5. Repeat 8 times.

Cautions and Comments

- Move with control. Don't rock up and down—that's cheating.
- Babies usually love this exercise, so try to fit it in whenever you sit down on the floor with your baby (you will see a tight tummy a lot faster).

Horsie Ride

Benefits

- Tones the buttocks and the vaginal muscles
- Strengthens gluteals, hamstrings, lumbar erector spinae, ankle and toe dorsiflexors, hip adductors, hip rotators
- Stretches iliopsoas muscle group and abdominalis muscles

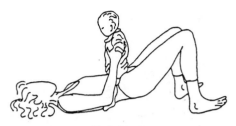

A. STARTING POSITION

Directions

1. Lie on your back with your knees bent and your feet flat on the floor, hip distance apart (Figure 13.8A).
2. Hold your baby in a sitting position just above your pubic bone (a small baby can lie on your tummy and chest).
3. Curl your pubic bone and tailbone under, bringing your hips and waist off the floor (Figure 13.8B). Squeeze your buttocks muscles.
4. Release your buttocks muscles and lower your hips slightly (not all the way to the floor).
5. Repeat squeezing and releasing 8 times.
6. Flex your toes off the floor and repeat the squeezing and releasing 8 times.
7. Separate your feet so that they are wider than your hips. Flex your feet.
8. Press your knees together, squeezing your buttocks (Figure 13.8C), then open your knees and release your buttocks (Figure 13.8D).
9. Repeat 16 times.

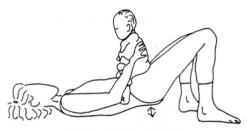

B. RAISING HIPS AND WAIST

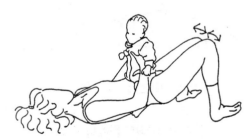

C. PRESSING KNEES TOGETHER

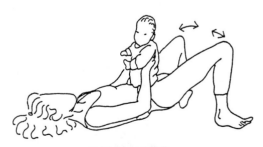

D. OPENING KNEES

Figure 13.8 Horsie Ride

Cautions and Comments

- Do not lower your hips down to the floor upon release.
- Do not bounce your hips up and down.

Flying Baby

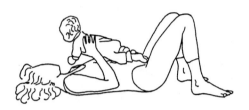

A. STARTING POSITION

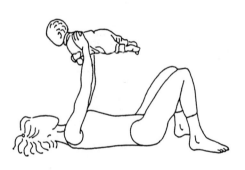

B. PRESSING BABY UP IN THE AIR

Figure 13.9   Flying Baby

Benefits

• Strengthens the chest area
• Strengthens pectoralis muscle group; serratus anterior, triceps brachii, and anterior deltoid muscles

Directions

1. Lie on your back with your knees bent and feet flat on the floor, hip distance apart.
2. Hold your baby close to your chest (Figure 13.9A).
3. Press the baby straight up into the air (Figure 13.9B), then lower him back to your chest.
4. Repeat 8 times.

Cautions and Comments

• Try to keep your baby's body parallel to yours.
• This is a good exercise for strengthening your baby's back and neck muscles.

Kiss-the-Baby Push-Ups

Benefits

- Strengthens arm, lower back, and abdominal muscles
- Strengthens pectoralis and abdominalis muscle groups; serratus anterior, triceps brachii, rectus abdominus, gluteals, and hamstrings

Directions

1. Begin on your hands and knees with your ankles crossed, knees bent, and your baby lying between your hands (Figure 13.10A). Your weight should be resting above your kneecaps.
2. Tuck your hips under so your shoulders, hips, and knees form a straight line. Your hands should be directly under your shoulders with the fingers angled slightly inward.
3. Inhale as you lower yourself down to kiss your baby (Figure 13.10B). Exhale as you push up.
4. Repeat 4-16 times.

Cautions and Comments

- Maintain proper alignment as you lower yourself.
- Start out by doing a few, then add one more push-up every other time you work out.

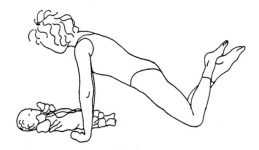

A. STARTING POSITION

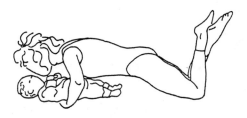

B. BENDING DOWN TO KISS BABY

Figure 13.10 Kiss-the-Baby Push-Ups

Baby Swings

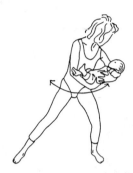

SWINGING BABY FROM SIDE TO SIDE

Figure 13.11   Baby Swings: Variation I

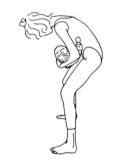

A. STARTING CRADLE POSITION

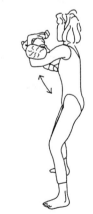

B. SWINGING BABY UP

Figure 13.12   Baby Swings: Variation II

Benefits

- Strengthens gastrocnemius; soleus, hip adductor, and pectoralis muscle groups; quadriceps, biceps brachii, and anterior deltoids
- Stretches hip adductor, gastrocnemius, and soleus muscle groups

Directions for Variation I

1. Stand with your feet approximately 3 feet apart and turned out slightly.
2. Hold your baby in a cradle or a sitting position.
3. Lunge right, then left, gently swinging baby from side to side (Figure 13.11).
4. Repeat 8 times.

Directions for Variation II

1. Stand with your feet approximately 3 feet apart, knees slightly bent.
2. Hold the baby in cradle position.
3. Round your back down, bringing the baby close to you (Figure 13.12A).
4. Swing the baby up (Figure 13.12B), then lower him back down.
5. Repeat 8 times.

Cautions and Comments

- Make sure your abdominal muscles are pulled in before you swing up.
- Remember to keep your knees bent and maintain a pelvic tilt.
- Very small babies might become startled during this exercise.
- Practice slowly and easily.

Standing Spinal Twist

Benefits

- Keeps the spine limber, which has a therapeutic effect on your nervous system
- Strengthens and stretches the cervical, thoracic, and lumbar erector spinae; obliques; quadriceps; gastrocnemius and soleus muscle groups; scapular and chest muscle groups (rhomboid, middle trapezius, pectorals)

Directions

1. Stand with your feet parallel and approximately 3 feet apart. Bend your knees slightly.
2. Rest your baby on your hip (Figure 13.13A).
3. Straighten your legs as you twist your spine, looking all the way around behind you (Figure 13.13B).
4. Pass through the starting position as you twist to the other side.
5. Repeat 4 times in each direction.

Cautions and Comments

- Be sure both hips are facing forward as you twist.
- Only your upper body should twist.

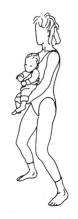

A. STARTING POSITION

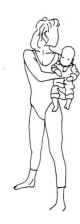

B. TWISTING UPPER BODY

Figure 13.13   Standing Spinal Twist

Side Stretch with Baby

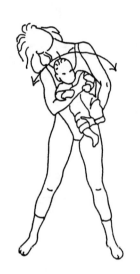

STRETCHING TO THE SIDES

Figure 13.14   Side Stretches

Benefits

• Stretches and tones the waist area
• Strengthens obliques, quadratus lumborum, upper trapezius, and lateral cervical muscles

Directions

1. Stand with your feet parallel and approximately 3 feet apart.
2. Hold your baby with his back against your chest/abdomen.
3. Stretch your upper body to the right twice, return to the starting position, then repeat to the left (Figure 13.14).
4. Repeat right and left 8 times.

Cautions and Comments

• Maintain proper body alignment by keeping your shoulders in line with your hips.
• Dropping your shoulders back will put strain on your lower back. Be careful.

Heel Lifts

Benefits

- Strengthens the calf, toe, and ankle muscles
- Stretches and strengthens quadriceps, ankle and toe dorsi flexors, gastrocnemius and soleus muscle groups

Directions

1. Stand with your feet approximately 3 feet apart, knees bent, and feet turned outward.
2. Lift your right heel, then lower it. Lift your left heel, then lower it (Figure 13.15).
3. Do 8-16 lifts with each heel.

Cautions and Comments

- Make sure you do not arch your lower back.
- Keep your shoulders directly over your hips.

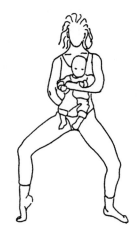

RAISING AND LOWERING HEELS

Figure 13.15 Heel Lifts

Exercise Routines for Daddy and Baby

Being a new dad certainly takes up a great deal of your time, but it is not wise (nor is it necessary) to eliminate leisure-time activities from your life. With the aid of a little creativity, your new baby can easily take part in some of your extra-curricular activities. Just as a new mom can involve her baby when she is doing shape-up exercises, a new dad can involve his new son or daughter in the stretching exercises that should precede or follow athletic activity. Proper stretching can help prevent injury as well as improve performance.

The exercises found in this section, though designed with dads in mind, can be effectively practiced by both dads and moms. You will find involving your baby in the following stretching exercises can be an enjoyable, worthwhile, and entertaining way to bond with your child.

Lateral Side Stretch

Benefits

- Stretches, warms, and revitalizes the muscles located on the sides of the body
- Tones and trims the waist, while releasing neck tension
- Stretches and strengthens oblique and transversus abdominalis, quadratus lumbar, thoraco-lumbar, erector spinae and fascia, latissimus dorsi, lateral and posterior cervical erector spinae, scaleni, hip abductors and adductors, iliotibial band, and tensor fascia latae

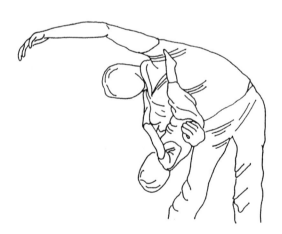

Figure 13.16   Lateral Side Stretch

Directions

1. Stand up straight with your legs about 3 feet apart, and place your child securely on your left hip.
2. Stretch your right arm straight up from your shoulder, keeping it close to your right ear.

3. Hold on to your child as you stretch over to your left side (Figure 13.16).
4. Hold without bouncing for as long as you wish, then return to the starting position.
5. Take an Abdominal Breath (page 17) and repeat on the other side.
6. Do 2-3 stretches on each side.

Cautions and Comments

• For an effective stretch, try keeping your top arm straight and as close to your ear as possible.
• Separating your feet an increased distance will add an additional stretch to the groin area.

Open "V" Stretch

Benefits

• Keeps arms firm and supple
• Helps trim the waist area
• Stretches and strengthens the gastrocnemius, soleus, hip adductor, and pectoralis muscle groups; the hamstrings, oblique and transversus abdominalis, thoraco erector spinae and fascia, latissimus dorsi, teres major, triceps brachii, and the lateral, posterior, cervical erector spinae

Directions

1. Sit on a mat with your legs in an open "V" position. Stretch your right arm down your right leg and grasp your toe. (If this is too difficult, hold your ankle instead.)
2. Stretch your left arm up into the air until it is parallel with your right arm (Figure 13.17).
3. Hold this position while talking to your child for as long as is comfortable.
4. Return to the starting position, take an Abdominal Breath (page 17), and repeat on the other side.
5. Stretch 3 times on each side.

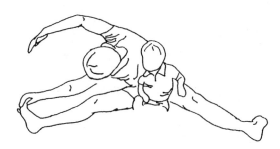

Figure 13.17 Open "V" Stretch

Cautions and Comments

• For the most effective stretch, *do not bounce* when in side-stretching position. Hold steady.
• For an increased stretch, place your left hand on your right hand.
• This is an excellent stretch before playing tennis or racquetball.

Abdominal / Shoulder Toners

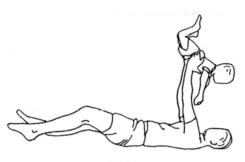

A. LIFTING BABY UP

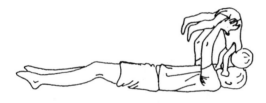

B. MOVING FORWARD AND BACK

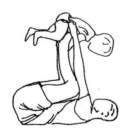

C. PLACING BABY ON FEET

Figure 13.18   Abdominal/Shoulder Toner
Sequence

Benefits

• Tones the legs and spine
• Stretches and strengthens pectoralis, iliopsoas, gastrocnemius, soleus, hip adductor, and the transversus and oblique abdominalis muscle group; triceps brachii, serratus anterior, lumbar erector spinae, quadriceps, and hamstrings

Directions

1. Lie on your back and place your child, tummy down, on your chest.
2. Holding the child with both hands, lift him in the air and move him from side to side and forward and back (Figures 13.18A and 13.18B).
3. Bend your knees to your chest and carefully place your child on your feet (Figure 13.18C).

4. Straighten your legs up in the air while holding on to your child's hands (Figure 13.18D). Hold this position for as long as is comfortable.

5. Move your baby from side to side before slowly lowering him down between your open legs (Figure 13.18E) and then onto your chest for a big hug (Figure 13.18F)!

6. Take a deep breath and relax.

Cautions and Comments

• It is advisable to practice this series with an older child.
• If you are not used to doing this type of stretch, it is advisable to go through the steps without your child for the first time.
• This is an enjoyable way to tone your abdominal muscles!

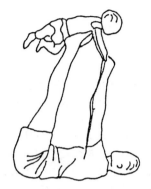

D. UP INTO THE AIR!

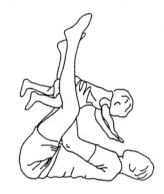

E. LOWERING BABY

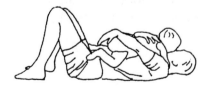

F. FATHER-BABY HUG

Shoulder/Thigh Toners

Benefits

- Eliminates tension, tiredness, and soreness from your shoulders, thighs, and calves
- Helps tone the abdominal area
- Stretches and strengthens rhomboideus, gastrocnemius, and soleus muscle groups; cervical, thoracic, and lumbar erector spinae; lower and mid trapezius muscles; serratus anterior; latissimus dorsi; gluteus maximus; and hamstring muscles

Directions

1. Sit on a mat with your legs together and straight out in front of you. Place your baby at your side.
2. Stretch your arms forward and place fingers on your toes (Figure 13.19). Feel the stretch across your shoulders and throughout your legs.
3. Increase the stretch by pointing your toes.
4. Hold this position for 30-60 seconds. Return to a sitting position and take an Abdominal Breath (page 17).

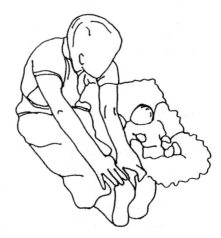

Figure 13.19   Shoulder/Thigh Toner

Cautions and Comments

- If you cannot reach your toes without bending your knees, place your hands on your ankles and bend your elbows out to the sides. This will give you a similar (but not as effective) stretch.
- With practice, you will find increased flexibility in your lower back and shoulders.

Calf/Thigh/Hip Toner

Benefits

- This an excellent post-running stretch
- Stretches and strengthens hip adductor, pectoralis, and iliopsoas muscle groups; rectus femoris, hip external rotators, gluteals

Directions

1. Sitting with your right leg bent behind you and your left heel as close to your groin as possible, place your child on top of your bent leg.
2. Pull your right heel as close to your hip as possible (Figure 13.20).
3. Hold the stretch for 30-60 seconds before repeating the stretch on the other side.

Cautions and Comments

- Do not bend your leg to the point of discomfort.
- If you have knee problems, be careful with this stretch.

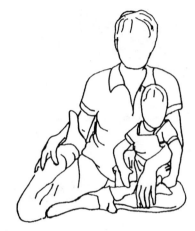

Figure 13.20   Calf/Thigh/Hip Toner

Weighted Legs

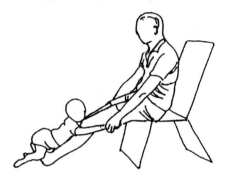

A. STARTING POSITION

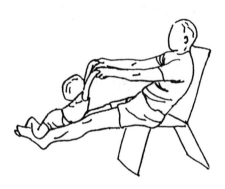

B. GIVING CHILD A RIDE

Figure 13.21   Weighted Legs

Benefits

- Tones the buttocks, legs, and abdomen
- Stretches and strengthens iliopsoas and quadricep muscle groups, and rectus abdominalis

Directions

1. Sit in a chair with your legs together and your knees locked. Place your child comfortably on your ankles (Figure 13.21A).
2. Lift both of your legs up into the air and give your child a ride (Figure 13.21B).
3. Hold your legs up as long as is comfortable, then lower them down.
4. Repeat 5-10 times.

Cautions and Comments

- You may want to finish this stretch well before your child does.
- With practice, you will be able to hold your child up for longer periods of time.

The Split

Benefits

- Is an excellent post-running stretch
- Stretches and strengthens iliopsoas, quadriceps, hamstring, gluteals, hip adductors, gastrocnemius, and soleus muscle groups; thoraco-lumbar spinae

Directions

1. Begin this stretch on your knees.
2. Extend your right leg out in front of you while leaning back on your left knee. Sit your child on your right ankle.
3. Stretch forward into a split (Figure 13.22), and hold for as long as is comfortable.
4. Repeat on the other side.

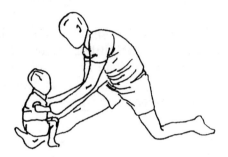

Figure 13.22   The Split

Cautions and Comments

- This is a very dynamic stretch and can be a little painful for those unused muscles. With practice, tight thighs and buttocks muscles will loosen up.
- Talk to your child as you stretch forward. This will maximize the time for each stretch.

Lower-Back Stretch

Benefits

- Warms, soothes, and strengthens the lower back
- Eliminates lower backaches
- Releases tension from the shoulders and arms
- Stretches and straightens hamstring attachments at gluteii, thoraco-lumbar erector spinae and fascia, mid-lower trapezii, rhomboids, cervical erector spinae, and upper trapezii

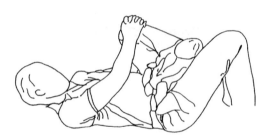

Figure 13.23   Lower-Back Stretch

Directions

1. Lie on your back with your knees bent and both feet flat on the mat, separated about 6 inches. Place the baby in a sitting position with his back against your thighs. Take a deep breath and exhale.
2. Bring your left knee to your chest and wrap both arms around it.
3. Press your knee as close to your chest as is comfortable, but be sure to keep your lower back flat on the mat (Figure 13.23).
4. Hold for 30-60 seconds.
5. Repeat 3-4 times on each side.

Cautions and Comments

- This is a great stretch to warm your lower back prior to athletic activity.
- You can add a neck stretch to this exercise by bringing your nose to your knee.

You may have your own favorite stretches that can easily be practiced while involving your child. Be inventive and create your own special series. *Stretching for Runners* and *Stretching for Athletes* are both excellent tapes on stretching (pages 309 and 310).

Family Stretches

One of the joys of having a family is sharing enjoyable activities together. Moving, stretching, and massaging as a family can become part of your new awareness of each other. Practice some of these family stretches and be aware of the good feelings that will result from this sharing time.

Family Back Massage

Benefits

- Massages and strengthens the lower back thereby eliminating back pain, tension, and fatigue
- Strengthens thoracic and lumbo-sacral erector spinae muscle groups
- Stretches hip adductors

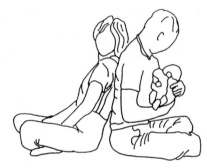

PUSHING BACK AND . . .

Directions

1. Sit back to back while one of you holds the baby.
2. Push against each other, forward and back (Figure 13.24).
3. Repeat as many times as you wish.

Cautions and Comments

- You can vary the feelings by pushing with different parts of your back. Experiment and find the variations you like best.
- This exercise can be addictive. Enjoy!

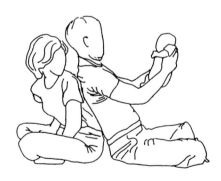

FORTH

Figure 13.24   Family Back Massage

Open "V" Family Stretch

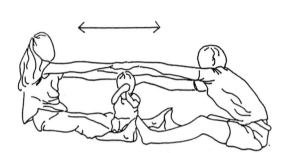

Figure 13.25   Open "V" Family Stretch

Benefits

- Loosens the lower back, thereby relieving backaches
- Tones and tightens the inner thighs
- Strengthens cervical, thoracic, and lumbar erector spinae muscles; pectoralis groups; serratus anterior; middle and lower trapezius
- Stretches thoraco lumbar fascia, erector spinae, gluteals, hip adductors, middle trapezius and rhomboideus muscle groups, serratus anterior and posterior muscle groups

Directions

1. Sit with your legs in an open "V" position facing your partner.
2. Place the soles of your feet together and place your baby between you.
3. Clasp hands with your partner and move forward and back (Figure 13.25).
4. Rock as far forward and back as you can.

Cautions and Comments

- You may discover one particular position that feels wonderful. If so, freeze and hold the stretch for a few seconds before moving again.
- Vary the speed while doing this exercise. Moving very fast or very slow is fun for a change of pace.

Family Baby Swing

Benefits

- For baby: strengthens and stretches spinal muscles and strengthens spinal extension; strengthens the arm and leg muscles
- For you: stretches thoracic lumbar fascia and erector spinae, quadriceps lumborium, hip muscles, transversus and oblique abdominalis muscles, wrists, and ankles
- Is fun for everyone

Directions

1. Stand and face one another while holding your child by his hands and feet.
2. Gently swing him from side to side (Figure 13.26).
3. Wait for waves of laughter.

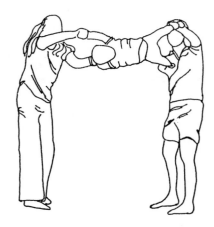

Figure 13.26   Family Baby Swing

Cautions and Comments

- This is excellent for improving your baby's balance and his spatial awareness.
- This exercise should be done with children over six months old.
- Only swing your child as high as he desires. This exercise should be fun, not frightening.
- Be careful not to pull too hard on your child; ligament structures in his wrists and ankles could be damaged.

CHAPTER FOURTEEN
Exercises Designed to Relieve Backaches

Throughout my second pregnancy I was plagued with a chronic backache. I assumed once I gave birth, the backache would disappear. I was totally wrong. Through attending a yoga class I discovered one has to strengthen and stretch one's lower- and middle-back muscles while realigning the spine in order to rid oneself of back pain. When I began working with new mothers, I found that many of them experienced tension and aching in their middle and upper backs from feeding and caring for their babies around the clock. Others complained of lower-back pain due to weak abdominal muscles.

Proper precautions have to be taken during the weeks and months after giving birth. Practicing self-massage plus incorporating daily stretching and strengthening for the lower-, middle-, and upper-back muscles should help relieve backaches. The exercises in this chapter are designed to do just that.

SENSIBLE TIPS ON PREVENTING BACKACHES AND BACK DAMAGE

- When sitting, make sure your lower spine and back are pressed well into the back of the chair. Use a small pillow against your lower back to hold your back upright. Remember to maintain good posture while sitting. Do not slouch in a soft chair or sit on any soft furniture that allows your knees to be higher than your hips.
- A backache can be the result of sleeping on a mattress that is too soft. If your mattress is too soft and you do not want to buy a new one, place a large piece of half-inch-thick plywood between the box spring and mattress for added back support. Many women find that water beds can be beneficial for eliminating backaches. Physical therapist Carl Mailhot suggests attaching a rolled-up towel around your waist with a safety pin or belt

- When getting out of bed, avoid twisting or turning with your knees apart. First, tighten your abdominal muscles, bend your knees, and roll onto your side. Next, push yourself up with your arms into a sitting position. Put both legs over the side of the bed, keep your knees together, and stand up.
- When standing up to do household jobs, such as washing the dishes or straightening drawers, put one foot up on a low stool or on the bottom shelf of a cupboard. This will help eliminate strain from your lower back and will help get your spine back into its proper alignment. If you don't have these options, gently bend your knees, pull in your abdomen, and tilt your pelvis back to line up with your hips and back.
- Protect your lower back by doing "low" household chores, such as bathing the baby, on your knees.
- Kneel or squat when picking things up off the floor. (See the inset on page 243 for the correct way to lift heavy things.)
- Make sure to choose a stroller or carriage with handles that are high enough to push without having to stoop forward.
- Choose a front or backpack carrier that holds your baby centrally, either in front or back. Make sure you chose one that is adjustable. A baby sling can also be helpful in easing back strain when carrying your baby, as well as a convenient device to use when breastfeeding (Figure 14.1).
- Your changing table should be just the right height for you. About waist level is recommended during the early months postpartum.

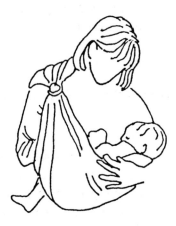

Figure 14.1   Baby Sling

When Lifting Toddlers and Other Heavy Objects

The following suggestions should be heeded in order to avoid back problems when lifting toddlers and other heavy objects:

- Before your lift, pull in on your abdominal muscles, tuck in your buttocks, and brace your pelvic floor.
- Keep your spine straight.
- Bring the object to be lifted close to your body.
- Test the weight of the object with your arms first—if it's too heavy to lift with both arms, you're going to need help. Kneel or squat down next to the object; using your stronger thigh muscles to bear most of the weight, slowly rise until you are standing (Figure 14.2).
- Never lift anything when bending or twisting to the side.
- When pushing or pulling any weight, make sure your knees are bent and mobile.

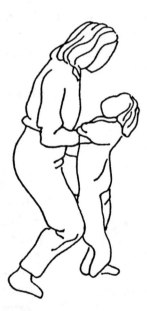

Figure 14.2   Correct Lifting Position

BACK-MASSAGING EXERCISES

The following massages are designed to prepare the lower and middle back for stretching by bringing blood and warmth to these areas. These massages should always precede and/or follow any strenuous stretching. Another good reason to do them—they feel terrific!

Lower-Back Massage with Baby

Benefits

- Warms, stimulates, and energizes the spine in preparation for more strenuous exercises
- Is very relaxing and can be performed during hectic times as a quick tension releaser and energizer
- Gives the baby an enjoyable ride
- Stretches thoracic and lumbar erector spinae muscle groups, multifedii, gluteus maximus, and quadriceps (except rectus femoris)

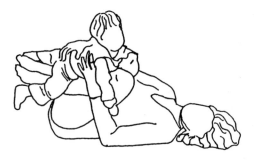

Figure 14.3 Lower-Back Massage with Baby

Directions

1. Lying on your back, bend your knees and bring them up to your chest.
2. Rest your baby's tummy on your shins.
3. Slowly rock from side to side, massaging your lower back while giving your baby a pleasant ride (Figure 14.3).
4. Keep massaging, breathing normally, for at least two minutes until you feel warmth in your lower-back area.

Cautions and Comments

- This important exercise should be used to massage the lower back after completing lower-back postures such as the Bridge (page 132) and the Shoulderstand (page 144).
- Always practice this exercise on a padded surface, never on a hard floor.
- Be careful not to rock too far to one side or you might roll over. With a minimum of practice you will be able to gauge your movements.

Pendulum Legs

Benefits

- Releases tension from the lower back
- Relieves lower backache
- Helps tone the thighs, waist, and buttocks
- Relaxes the entire body
- Stretches and strengthens thoracolumbar, lumbar pelvic muscles and fascia, quadratus lumborum, gluteals, hip rotators, hip abductors and adductors

Directions

1. Lie on your back with your baby on your chest. Bend both legs at the knee, bring them together, and drop them to one side (Figure 14.4). They should be flat on the floor and as close to your body as is comfortable.
2. Move your legs from side to side like a pendulum.
3. Eventually let your legs fall to one side for 5-10 seconds. Repeat on the other side.
4. Keep moving your legs in a pendulum motion until your lower back feels warm and relaxed.
5. Finish with 1-2 Abdominal Breaths (page 17).

Cautions and Comments

- You do not have to keep your feet on the ground as you move your legs from side to side.

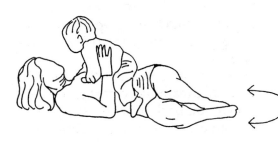

Figure 14.4   Pendulum Legs

Universal Pose

See page 150 for directions.

Back-Stretching Exercises

The Cobra

Benefits for All Cobra Variations

- Strengthens the spine and eliminates tension, especially in the middle and lower back
- Helps realign vertebrae
- Helps relieve lower backache
- Firms and minimizes buttocks area
- Stretches and strengthens pectoral muscles and fascia; anterior cervical, thoracic, lumbar erector-spinae; abdominal, trapezii, rhomboideus muscle groups; triceps brachii; wrist, forearm, and finger flexors

Directions for the Low Cobra (Variation I)

1. Lie on your stomach with your hands at your sides and your legs straight. Rotate your legs inward so that your big toes face one another.
2. Place the baby in front of or beside you.

3. Place your hands, palms down, on the floor under your shoulders. Keep your elbows close to your body and your chin in the center of the mat.
4. Slowly raise your head (only) up into the air while stretching your chin up toward the ceiling. Hold for 5-10 seconds.
5. Now raise your shoulders, using your mid-back muscles rather than your arms (Figure 14.5). Be careful not to overextend yourself.
6. Stretch your chin up toward the ceiling and stretch your spine without using your arms. Use your arms for balance.
7. Hold this stretched position for 5-30 seconds, breathing normally, and then slowly roll back down to the mat or continue up into a High Cobra (Variation II).
8. If you come down, put your head to the side and take 1-2 Abdominal Breaths (page 17) and relax.

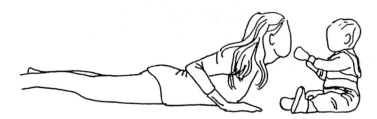

Figure 14.5   Low Cobra

Directions for the High Cobra (Variation II)

1. You can begin the High Cobra by following directions 1 and 2 of the Low Cobra, or after holding a Low Cobra for 10-15 seconds.
2. Lift the trunk of your body as high into the air as possible (Figure 14.6).
3. Reach your chin up to the ceiling for maximum stretch.
4. Make sure your pelvic area is on the mat and your back is arched as far back as is comfortable. If you cannot keep your pelvic area on the mat, either move your hands away from you or place a small pillow under your pelvis for support.
5. Hold stretch for 5-30 seconds, then roll back down with control, taking at least 15 seconds, lowering your head last.
6. Turn your head to the side, take 1-2 Abdominal Breaths (page 17), and relax.

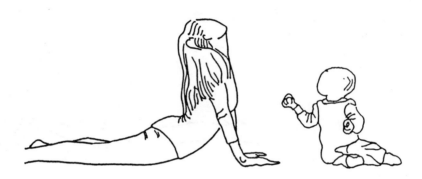

Figure 14.6 High Cobra

Directions for the Triangle Cobra (Variation III)

1. Lie on your stomach and place your hands, palms down, under your chin. Your fingers should be touching and your elbows should be out to the sides (Figure 14.7A).
2. Raise your head up, followed by your shoulders, without using your arms. Raise up as high as you can.
3. Stretch your chin toward the ceiling and hold this position for 10-30 seconds while breathing normally.
4. Push on your hands and raise up as high as you can, arching your back and keeping your pelvis on the mat (Figure 14.7B). Your arms may still be somewhat bent.

5. Hold for 10-30 seconds, breathing normally, then roll down slowly, taking 15 seconds for the descent. Keep your chin up as you roll down. Your head should be last to come down.

6. Turn your head to the side, take 1-2 Abdominal Breaths (page 17), and relax.

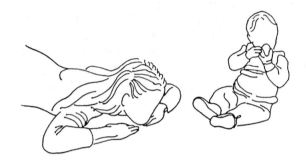

A. STARTING POSITION

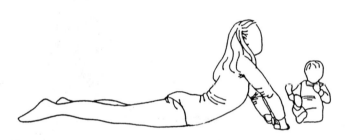

B. ARCHING UP

Figure 14.7   Triangle Cobra

Cautions and Comments for All Cobra Variations

• Those with neck or lower-back pain should approach this exercise very carefully. Cobras can be painful if you have a weak lower back. If this is your case, you can still practice Cobras, just don't stretch up so high that you feel pain. Stretch to the edge of pain, not into it.

• The High Cobra should be practiced only after the Low Cobra can be comfortably completed.

• If you are breastfeeding, be sure to place a foam pad under your breasts before doing Cobras. It will increase your comfort.

• Make sure you are moving one vertebra at a time. This will massage your spine.

• Try timing your breathing with the cobra movements. Take a deep Abdominal Breath with the press-up, and exhale as you roll down slowly, one vertebra at a time.

• With daily practice, these exercises can help relieve lower and mid backaches while giving you pep and energy.

• Moving slowly into and out of the Cobras is important for their effectiveness.

Pelvic-Tilt Wall Stretch

Benefits

- Tones the abdominal muscles
- Helps relieve lower backache
- Stretches lumbo-pelvic erector spinae muscles, pectoral muscles and fascia
- Strengthens oblique and transverse abdominalis muscle groups; deep iliopsoas muscle groups; pelvic floor muscles (when combined with the Squeeze, page 122, and Kegels, page 104); lower and middle trapezii muscles

Directions

1. Stand next to a wall with your feet about 12 inches apart. Press your lower back into the wall.
2. Extend your arms up the wall, making sure they remain in contact with the wall (Figure 14.8).
3. Feel the stretch in your lower back as you breathe. Hold 30-60 seconds.
4. Release and repeat 3 times.

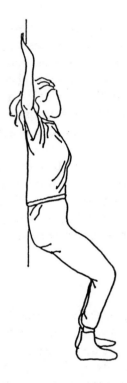

Figure 14.8 Pelvic-Tilt Wall Stretch

Cautions and Comments

- You may feel instant relief for your lower backache after this pelvic tilt.
- Allow your knees to unlock and gently bend during this exercise.
- Try to keep your head, neck, and shoulders against the wall.

Back Stretcher

Benefits

- Stretches the entire body but is particularly effective for the mid-upper back
- Tones the arms, back, thighs, and calves
- Strengthens and tones all portions of the trapezii muscles especially the lower trapezii, the rhomboideus muscle group, the cervical and thoracic erector spinae, latissimus dorsi, the deltoideus muscle groups, and the triceps muscles
- Stretches the gastrocnemius and soleus muscles, the gluteus maximus, the lumbar erector spinae, the pectoralis muscles, the latissimus dorsi, and the anterior chest wall fascia

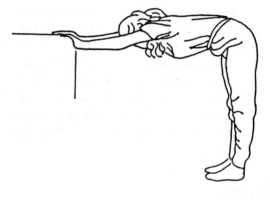

Figure 14.9   Back Stretcher

Directions

1. Standing directly in front of, place your hands on a wall. Your hands should be shoulder-distance apart.
2. Back away from the wall until you begin to feel a stretch in your back, arms, and thighs (Figure 14.9).
3. Pull in your abdominal muscles as you extend your spine and lengthen the front of your body.
4. Feel the stretch in your back, arms, and shoulders as well as in your thighs as you pull backward a bit, holding the position. Your hips should be in line with your feet.
5. Hold the stretch for 30 seconds to 2 minutes while breathing normally.
6. Walk back to the starting position and take an Abdominal Breath (page 17).
7. Repeat 4-5 times.

Cautions and Comments

- Instead of a wall, you can perform this stretch while holding on to a counter or crib.
- This is an effective stretch to do after you have been holding your baby for a while. It will help release the tension in your upper back and shoulders, which can eventually turn into a stiff neck or headache.
- For additional abdominal tightening, exhale completely while in stretched position, pull in your tummy, and hold for 10-30 seconds.
- To relieve neck tightness, stretch your chin up toward the ceiling while holding the stretched position.

Chest Expander

Benefits

- Releases tension and tightness in the neck, shoulders, and upper and lower back while strengthening these areas
- Develops and strengthens the muscles that support the breasts
- Expands the lung and chest area for increased breathing capacity
- Strengthens middle trapezius and rhomboideus muscle groups, thoracic erector spinae muscles, latissimus dorsi/teres major group; isometrically strengthens abdominal muscles
- Stretches upper trapezius, pectoralis major and minor muscle groups and scalenus muscle group.

Directions

1. Sit in a cross-legged position and clasp your hands behind your back with your palms facing up.
2. Inhale and gently raise your clasped hands as high as you can, then exhale and lower them back down to your buttocks (Figure 14.10).
3. Repeat this movement 3-4 times to warm and limber your chest muscles.
4. Then, breathing normally, raise your clasped hands behind you and hold for 30 seconds to 2 minutes.
5. Release and take 1-2 Abdominal Breaths (page 17).

Cautions and Comments

- This exercise stretches many sets of muscles in your chest and back in ways they are not used to. As a result, you may find resistance to these movements when you first begin to practice. Keep practicing, though. Eventually, you will notice increased flexibility in your upper body.
- To increase the stretch across your chest and shoulders, try some of the clasped hand movements with your palms touching and thumbs together.
- If you can't clasp your hands because of tightness, hold a broomstick or a dowel behind your back and lift it away from your buttocks.
- Don't let your shoulders roll down and forward. Keep your chest and breastbone up.

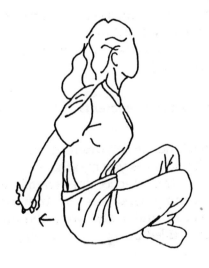

Figure 14.10   Chest Expander

Sitting Wall Stretch

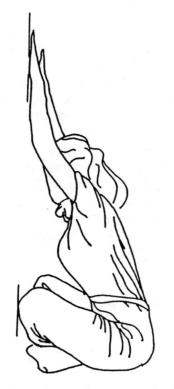

Figure 14.11   Sitting Wall Stretch

Benefits

- Releases tension from the mid-upper back
- Stretches lower trapezii, latissimus dorsi/teres major muscle group, thoraco-lumbar erector spinae, pectoralis muscles and fascia
- Strengthens mid and cervical-thoracic erector spinae; isometrically strengthens abdominals, hip adductors, and hip rotators

Directions

1. Sit in a cross-legged position facing a wall. Stretch your arms up and place your hands on the wall. (Figure 14.11.) Feel an invigorating stretch across your shoulders.
2. Breathe normally and hold the stretch 30 seconds to 2 minutes.
3. Release and take 1-2 Abdominal Breaths (page 17).

Cautions and Comments

- Feel the tension draining out of your shoulders as you breathe.
- You can practice this stretch while standing. Make sure your buttocks are tucked under and your abdominals are pulled in.

CHAPTER FIFTEEN

Exercise and Your Daily Routine

Did you ever realize that much of the time you spend feeding or taking care of your baby is a natural time to exercise? While breastfeeding or bottle-feeding, there are some wonderful ways to breathe as well as to practice minimal-movement exercises.

Also, since you are spending a great deal of time near your baby's crib, it makes sense to use the crib for assistance in doing some enjoyable stretches. You can easily talk to and interact with your baby while practicing (he may eventually conclude that his mommy is a ballerina). The added bonus is knowing you are tightening and toning your body as well as putting on a "performance." Try to incorporate at least one "crib stretcher" into your daily routine.

WHILE FEEDING THE BABY . . .

Eye Exercises

Benefits

- Help strengthen eye muscles
- Release tension and tiredness from your eyes
- Help relieve headaches
- Are very relaxing, and thereby enhance the feeding situation

Directions

1. Sit in a comfortable position with your back well supported, and begin to feed your baby.
2. Take 1-2 Abdominal Breaths (page 17).
3. Without moving your head, move your eyes as far to the right as you are able.

Then move them to the left (Figure 15.1A).

4. Move your eyes right and left 5 times, holding each movement for 1 second.
5. Close your eyes and take a deep breath.
6. Now, look up to the ceiling, then down to the floor (Figure 15.1B).
7. Move your eyes up and down 5 times, holding each movement for 1 second.
8. Close your eyes and take a deep breath.
9. If your eyes are not too tired, circle them 3 times clockwise and 3 times counterclockwise.
10. Close your eyes and relax.
11. If you have a free hand, place it over your eyes to induce a relaxed feeling.
12. Take several deep breaths and relax for several moments.

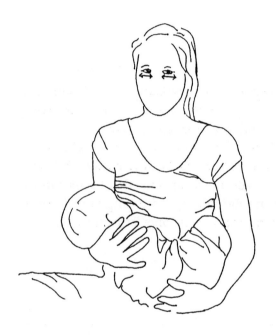

MOVING EYES RIGHT AND LEFT

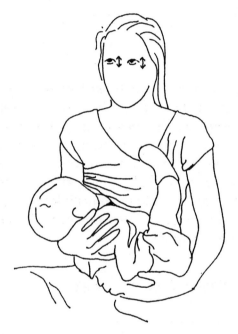

MOVING EYES UP AND DOWN

Figure 15.1   Eye Exercises

Cautions and Comments

• Since your baby was born, you have been using your eyes a lot more. As a result, your eye muscles can tire causing eyestrain. Eyestrain is a common cause of headaches.
• You can add other eye movements to the ones described above such as diagonals or half-circles.
• Take several moments for resting your eyes after a session. You may want to have a warm washcloth handy to place over your eyes.

Breathing Exercises

It is important to remember that you can enhance your baby's feeding experience by bringing yourself into a calm, relaxed state. The following breaths should be the most helpful to you during feedings:

- Abdominal Breath, page 17
- 2:8:4 Breath, page 18
- Alternate-Nostril Breath with Retention, page 18
- Tapus Heating Breath, page 105
- Energizing Single-Nostril Breath, page 22

Extremely active breaths are not on this list because they may disturb the baby and draw his attention away from eating. Complete as many rounds of the breaths mentioned as you can. The calmness they should bring you can be passed on to your baby, enhancing your relationship.

Neck Smiles

Complete directions found on page 166. These exercises can easily be performed while feeding your baby.

Kegels

Complete directions found on page 104. Practice at least one set of Kegels while nursing or bottle-feeding.

Abdominal Lift

Complete directions found on page 139. Do these while sitting cross-legged when feeding your baby.

WHILE STANDING AT THE CRIB...

Waist Stretch

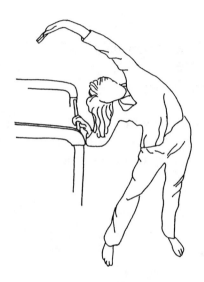

Figure 15.2   Waist Stretch

Benefits

- Tones and trims the waist and arms while releasing neck tension
- Provides an energizing stretch for each side of the body
- Stretches and strengthens oblique and transversus abdominalis, quadratus lumbar, thoraco-lumbar, latissimus dorsi, lateral and posterior cervical erector spinae, scalenii, hip abductors and adductors, iliotibial band, and tensor fascia latae

Directions

1. Stand with your right side a few inches from the crib and your feet about 12 inches apart.
2. Grasp the top of the crib with your right hand while bringing your left arm up above your head, palm facing down (Figure 15.2).
3. Maximize this stretch while breathing normally. Hold this posture for 5-30 seconds.
4. Slowly lower your arm, take 1-2 Abdominal Breaths (page 17), and repeat the same movement on the other side.

Cautions and Comments

- To maximize neck tension, relax your neck muscles once you are in the stretched position.
- Stretch over and talk to your baby as you hold this position.

Single Leg Lifts

Benefits

- Helps reduce hips and thighs
- Strengthens the lower back, minimizing backaches
- Helps make legs more shapely
- Stretches and strengthens lumbar erector spinae, gluteii, hamstrings and quadriceps; hip adductor and gastrocnemius muscle groups

Directions for Variation I

1. Stand about 12 inches away from the side of the crib and rest both hands on the crib rail.
2. Shift all of your weight to your right leg and extend your left leg up behind you as far as you can (Figure 15.3). Keep this extended leg straight.
3. Bend forward a bit and talk to your baby.
4. Lower your extended leg slowly and with control.
5. Take 1-2 Abdominal Breaths (page 17).
6. Repeat movements with the other leg.
7. Do 3-4 lifts with each leg.

Directions for Variation II

1. Follow steps 1 and 2 from Variation I, then move your extended leg as far to one side as is comfortable. Hold for 5-30 seconds.
2. Return leg to center and lower it slowly to the floor.
3. Take 1-2 Abdominal Breaths (page 17).
4. Repeat movements with your other leg.
5. Do 3-4 lifts with each leg.

Cautions and Comments

- If you feel any pain in your lower back, move your extended leg closer to the floor.
- Bending forward closer to the crib rail will help raise your back leg higher.
- This is an effective way to eliminate morning stiffness during your first visit to the baby's crib.
- Play peek-a-boo during this stretch.

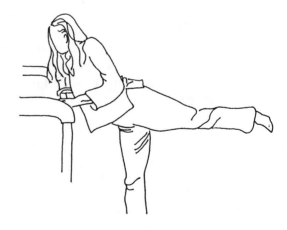

Figure 15.3 Single Leg Lift

Crib Squats

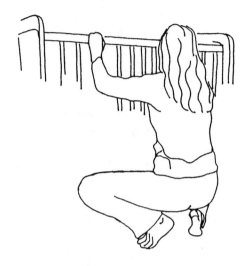

Figure 15.4   Crib Squat

Benefits

- Helps tighten the buttocks, hips, and thighs
- Helps prevent varicose veins
- Is a tension releaser
- Helps improve bodily elimination by stimulating the intestines
- Stretches and strengthens lumbar erector spinae; hip adductors, abductors and abdominalis muscle groups

Directions

1. Stand about 12 inches from the crib while loosely holding the crib rail with both hands.
2. Slowly bend your knees and go down into a squat on your toes. Try to keep your head up and spine straight (Figure 15.4).
3. Hold this stretch, breathing normally, for 5-30 seconds.
4. Return to the starting position while contracting your pelvic floor muscles.
5. Take 1-2 Abdominal Breaths (page 17) and repeat 2 times.

Cautions and Comments

- Your episiotomy should be completely healed (usually 2-3 weeks postpartum) before practicing crib squats.
- If this posture hurts your knees, do not practice it.

CHAPTER SIXTEEN

Baby Massage and Acupressure

*The mother of three healthy children
is more of an expert
on infant health
than the best doctor*

Oriental Proverb

Babies feel simply wonderful! Their skin is smooth, soft, and warm. They enjoy being soothed and touched; when held, they almost seem to mold themselves to you. Massaging your baby as part of a daily routine (if there is such a thing when you have a new baby) will give you and your baby mutual pleasure. If you have used any of the self- or partner-massage techniques found in Chapter Seven, then you are well-aware of the pleasure and relaxation that can be derived from massage. Massaging your baby regularly is a most effective bonding technique. Gentle, soothing words spoken to your baby along with eye and skin contact work together to enhance the special bond that connects you to your precious child. This experience provides the security of being loved and cared for in a relaxing, tension-free setting. You and your baby will look forward to this mutually satisfying activity.

The first section of this chapter deals with techniques for massaging your baby. Acupressure for your baby is discussed in the second half of this chapter. Basic acupressure techniques are given as a means to help relieve some common baby problems.

Baby Massage

Your baby's skin is his first means of communication with the outside world. All of your baby's sensors are vulnerable since he has not yet been conditioned to respond to stimulation in any certain way. Through a smooth, even, gentle massage technique, you can give your child very pleasurable sensations while sharing a uniquely loving time together. Often a massage will calm down a fussy baby so he can fall asleep.

Massage Guidelines

• Choose a warm, quiet place for giving the massage.

• Babies should be given a full body massage as soon as possible, for it helps encourage a general calmness. Colic can also be better controlled.

• As massage stimulation can cause spitting up, it is best to give a massage when the baby has an empty stomach. Covering your lap with a large, thick towel is also advisable.

• Generally, the best times for massage are early in the morning and before bed in the evening.

• A massage should last from ten to twenty minutes.

• Your baby's head should be shaded if you are massaging him in the sun.

• Use a heated oil or corn starch for lubrication. Baby oil is mineral oil and *should not* be used. Mineral oil is absorbed into the baby's skin where it clogs pores and depletes moisture. Almond oil, sesame oil, and baby lotion are preferable. Corn starch can also be used, which is especially good during hot weather.

• It is best to start the massage with the baby's arms or legs rather than his chest. This is so the baby is gradually introduced to the intimacy of the massage.*

---

*According to Vimala Schneider McClure, author of *Infant Massage: A Handbook for Loving Parents,* and Rebecca Goldstein, Certified Infant Massage Specialist.

Baby Massage Procedure

Directions

1. Begin by leaning back comfortably against a pile of cushions. Lean against a wall if this is more comfortable for you.
2. Place the baby, face up, on top of your extended legs (Figure 16.1). If you prefer, you can sit cross-legged with your baby lying on his back in front of you on a blanket or towel. Make sure you are comfortable.
3. Pour a bit of oil in your hands and rub them together to warm them up.
4. Roll your baby on to his right side a bit and begin the massage with his left arm. Hold on to his left wrist with your left hand and raise his arm.
5. Gently encircle his left shoulder with your right hand and, using a "milking" motion, slowly move your hand up the baby's arm until you have reached his hand (Figure 16.2).
6. Next, use both hands together in a twisting motion and work down from the baby's shoulder to his wrist. Massage and circle his wrist gently. Uncurl his fingers and massage his palms. Repeat several times.
7. Roll the baby onto his other side and repeat this procedure with his right arm.
8. Add a little more oil in your hands. Place your palms on the baby's chest and begin spreading the oil. Start at the center of his chest and spread your palms out to the sides. Repeat this motion several times, using gentle, fluid strokes (Figure 16.3). Do this until his chest is well-oiled.

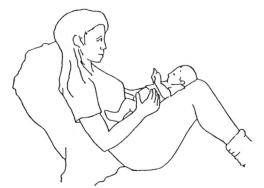

Figure 16.1 Starting Position

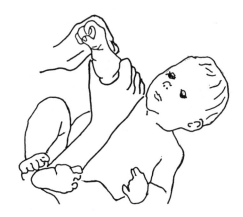

Figure 16.2 "Milking" Baby's Arm

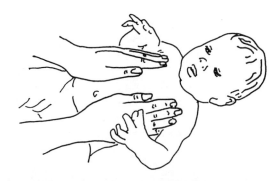

Figure 16.3 Spreading Oil on Chest

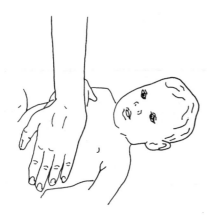

Figure 16.4   Hip-to-Shoulder Movement

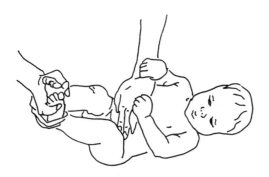

Figure 16.5   Massaging Tummy

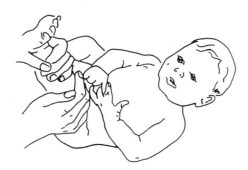

Figure 16.6   "Milking" Baby's Leg

9.   Using only one hand, place your palm on the baby's hip and tummy and move your palm up toward the baby's opposite shoulder (Figure 16.4). As soon as your palm reaches his shoulder, repeat the same motion with your other hand on the baby's other side. Keep these movements fluid as you cross and re-cross the baby's chest. Keep a slow, natural rhythm as you work.

10.   Next, massage the baby's tummy using both hands with alternating movements. These movements may stimulate digestion, resulting in a possible bowel movement or the passing of urine. To increase the relaxation of the tummy area, hold the baby's legs upward as you massage with the right (Figure 16.5). This will enable you to deepen the massage.

11.   Now, "milk" the baby's legs (Figure 16.6) using the same strokes that were used in Step 5. Use the palm of your hand to massage the bottom of his feet (you can use your thumbs, as well, if the baby is not ticklish). Gently massage the center of his feet for energy and tension release.

12.   Turn the baby over and lie him on his tummy with his head turned to the side. Rub more oil on your hands and use both hands to alternately massage his back. Do not use much pressure, rather just relax and let the movements flow freely. Place your thumbs on either side of his spine and gently move them out to the sides (Figure 16.7).

13.   Using two fingers, massage the baby's neck and shoulders using a back-and-forth motion (Figure 16.8).

14.   Hold the baby's buttocks firmly with your right hand as you use your left

hand to move slowly and consciously down his back. When you get to the buttocks, grasp the baby's feet (or under his knees) with your right hand while continuing to move your left hand down his legs to his feet (Figure 16.9). Repeat this movement in one long, continuous stroke.

15. Turn the baby over on his back. Massage his forehead using your fingertips. Start at the center of his forehead and massage down to his temples (Figure 16.10). Using your thumbs, massage either side of his nose, on his cheeks, and near his mouth. Some babies don't care for facial massage. You can simply stroke the area instead.

16. Finish by massaging the baby's scalp. Massaging the scalp is often an effective way to soothe a fussy baby. Effleurage or barely touching the baby with your fingers from his head to his toes can also be very pleasurable.

17. Using a soft towel, gently wipe off any excess oil or powder from the baby. Dress him and put him in for a nap. You should take one, too!

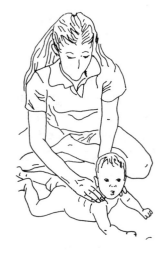

Figure 16.8 Massaging Neck and Shoulders

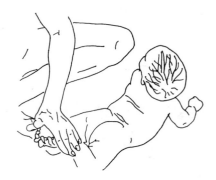

Figure 16.9 Massaging from Head to Toe

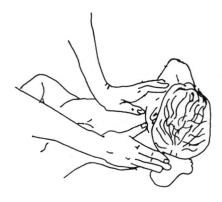

Figure 16.7 Massaging Back

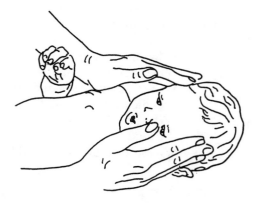

Figure 16.10 Massaging Baby's Face

Baby Acupressure

Shiatsu or *finger acupressure* is a therapy developed by the ancient Chinese. It consists of applying pressure to designated points on the skin's surface. These points, it is believed, can help heal certain diseases, restore specific organs to normal health, stop and/or prevent pain, stimulate deep-healing relaxation, and stimulate the body's own healing powers. These designated acupressure points connect the sense organs, tissues, upper and lower extremities, joints, and internal organs by means of channels or *meridians.* This explains why applying pressure to one area can affect another area far from the point of pressure.

Applying gentle finger acupressure can become a part of your daily routine to help balance the flow of your baby's energy. It can also be an extremely helpful tool in preventing an illness if applied when a symptom first begins to appear. It is, however, important to note that finger acupressure is *never* a cure. It should only be used as supplemental therapy and should *not* be a substitute for conventional care from your baby's pediatrician.

Applying Acupressure to Your Baby

According to Wataru Ohashi, shiatsu teacher and author of *Touch for Love: Shiatsu For Your Baby*, it is safe to use the pressure points found in this chapter as soon as your newborn's navel is healed. Keep the following points in mind when applying finger pressure to your child:

- Always use very light and gentle pressure. As your baby grows, you can gradually apply somewhat "heavier" pressure.
- When applying pressure, position the ball of your fingertip or thumb perpendicular to the area being treated.
- When applying pressure, a light circular movement or a jiggling motion can be used.
- Pressure should be applied from five to seven seconds on each spot.

ACUPRESSURE GUIDELINES

• Never apply acupressure on a baby with a cardiac condition.

• Avoid working on skin contusions, scars, or infected areas.

• Make sure the room is warm.

• Keep your hands clean and warm.

• It is important to keep your nails smooth and trimmed (just past the tip of your finger).

• Never work on a baby when he has a full stomach or an empty stomach. Your baby should be in an alert, playful state.

• Stop treatment if the baby becomes cranky, if the symptom is being aggravated, or if no relief is observed within a few minutes.

• Before beginning, put on some relaxing music (see page 310 for suggestions).

• Make sure you are in a relaxed, comfortable position that enables you to easily reach the entire length of your child's body.

• If you are applying acupressure on your child while he is lying on the floor, support your back with a pillow against a wall. Sit on a small cushion or a folded towel.

• Loosen any tight clothing you may be wearing. Take off your shoes.

• Always support or hold your baby gently with one hand while applying pressure with the other. Always keep at least one hand on the baby at all times.

Specific Baby Acupressure Points*

Applying acupressure to the following pressure points can help relieve the specific ailments indicated. These points can be safely used on children as well as on adults. As mentioned before, finger acupressure is considered a supplemental therapy and should never be used as a substitute for conventional care from your baby's doctor.

---

*After extensive research by Grace Burkhardt, RN, PPF instructor, and shiatsu practitioner, the pressure points presented here have been selected as most useful for your baby.

PRESSURE POINT #1

Uses For

- Sore throat
- Tonsillitis
- Fever
- Stuffy nose
- Toothache

Location

Found on the back of the hand between the bones of the thumb and index finger (see Figure 16.11).

Technique

Use the tip of your thumb to press firmly but gently on the pressure point for 5-7 seconds. Your thumb should be against the bone of the index finger.

PRESSURE POINT #2

Uses For

- General cold symptoms
- Cold with high fever
- Sore throat

Location

Found at the bottom *outside* corner of the thumbnail at the cuticle line (see Figure 16.12).

Technique

Use the tip of your finger to apply firm, steady pressure for 5-7 seconds.

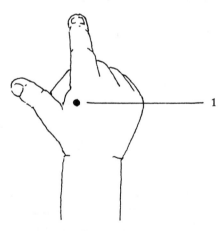

Figure 16.11   Pressure Point #1

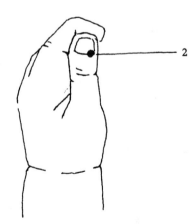

Figure 16.12   Pressure Point #2

PRESSURE POINT #3

Uses For

- Cold with cough

Location

On the top of the breastbone (see Figure 16.13).

Technique

Use your index finger to press inward, then massage downward into the notch at the top of the breastbone for 5-7 seconds.

PRESSURE POINT #4

Uses For

- Any stomach or abdominal problem

Location

Along the midline of the abdomen between the bottom of the breastbone and the bellybutton (see Figure 16.13).

Technique

On a hard surface, lie the baby on his back. Use your thumb to lightly massage inward at the pressure point for 5-7 seconds.

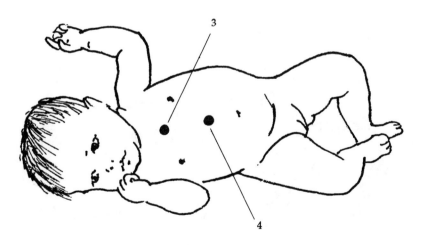

Figure 16.13 Pressure Points #3 and #4

PRESSURE POINT #5

Uses For

•Any stomach or abdominal problem

Location

Found just below the bellybutton (see Figure 16.13A).

Technique

On a hard surface, lie the baby on his back. Use your thumb to lightly massage inward at the pressure point for 5-7 seconds.

PRESSURE POINT #6

Uses For

•Constipation

Location

Found midway between the bellybutton and the pubic bone (see Figure 16.13A).

Technique

On a hard surface, lie the baby on his back. Use your thumb to lightly massage inward at the pressure point for 5-7 seconds.

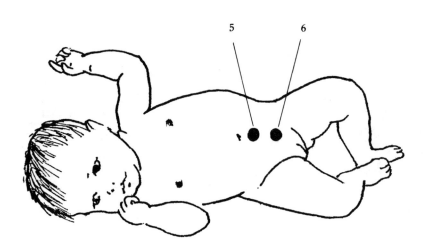

Figure 16.13A   Pressure Points #5 and #6

PRESSURE POINT #7

Uses For

- General cold symptoms
- Cold with fever
- Any breathing problem

Location

Found between the last cervical (neck) vertebra and the first thoracic (chest) vertebra (see Figure 16.14).

Technique

On a hard surface, position the baby on his stomach. Bend his head slightly forward. Use the tip of your index finger to apply light pressure while gently massaging for 5-7 seconds.

PRESSURE POINT #8

Uses For

- Cough
- Any lung or breathing problem

Location

Found on either side of the upper spine (see Figure 16.14).

Technique

Use the ball of your thumb to apply light pressure while gently massaging for 5-7 seconds.

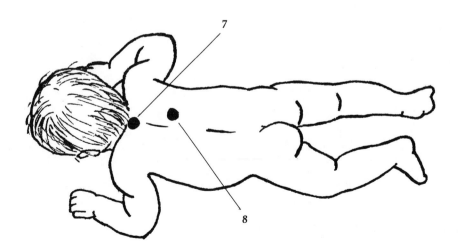

Figure 16.14 Pressure Points #7 and #8

CHAPTER SEVENTEEN
Baby Movement Program

More learning takes place during the first year of a baby's life than at any other time. It is a time of significant advances in the senses of sight, touch, and hearing as well as in the development of fine motor skills. It is when a baby's hand-eye coordination begins; it marks the onset of vocalization and the beginning stages of a baby's self-image. Babies whose muscles and senses are stimulated become more receptive to their surroundings.

A variety of fun activities with your baby can advance his natural developmental processes. These playful activities help stimulate the muscles and the senses while promoting a bond between you and your child. When you take an active part in your child's play, your presence creates positive feedback, and your child will feel motivated and secure enough to try new experiences.

For stimulating your baby's senses, use brightly colored toys made of various materials and textures. Allow your baby to visually track or follow colors, patterns, and shapes. Toys that create sounds or musical notes help develop auditory discrimination. Because infants are familiar with their parent's voices from life in the womb, they naturally enjoy hearing their parent's voices and observing adult faces. Singing, rhythmic chanting (as found when reciting nursery rhymes), and lots of eye contact with your baby are all extremely important in the development of rhythm and language, plus listening skills.

ADVANTAGES OF MOVEMENT PROGRAMS

Studies have shown that children in movement programs generally talk earlier, have better appetites, sleep more soundly, and experience greater acceleration in their motor development than those children who are not exercised. Infant movements accelerate motor development, coordination, and agility while increasing flexibility and strength. Since babies love to move and explore, the baby movements in this chapter will naturally cater to their needs. Exercising your baby will also help in the release of any stored tensions. You and your baby will enjoy the baby movement program found in this chapter.

GUIDELINES FOR MOVEMENT SESSIONS

- Before starting a movement program, discuss it with your baby's doctor. They are not recommended for all babies.
- Always place your baby on a soft surface such as a blanket that has been folded into a cushion.
- *Never* practice baby movements on a table, chair, or any other elevated surface for the baby could accidentally fall.
- Practice sessions with your baby should be no longer than twenty minutes. Do not practice more than two sessions in a day.
- If your baby cries or does not seem to be enjoying the session, simply stop.
- Make sure your baby is physically comfortable and happy.
- Be aware of your baby's responses while doing movements. A smile is a good indication that all is well.
- Be sensitive to your baby's needs. Do not exercise a hungry, tired, or ill baby. Do not practice with a baby as soon as he wakes up.
- Never do too much with the baby.
- Do not force limbs or torso into any uncomfortable position. Tune into and work with your child.
- Include lots of hugs and kisses in every movement session.
- Always start with joints that are closest to the baby's trunk. For example, loosen his shoulders before moving his elbows and his elbows before moving his hands.
- Move gently, guiding your baby's movements without force or quickness. This form of interaction should be playful, not mechanical.
- Sing to your baby during these sessions. The *Shape Up With Baby* audio cassette (page 309) provides the exercises found in this chapter with singing.

POSITIVE PARENTING FITNESS BABY MOVEMENT PROGRAM

This baby movement program is a basic program geared toward the first six to eight months of your baby's life. After a few sessions, your baby will begin to look forward to them. Each session builds on and strengthens the framework of intimacy, affection, and trust between you.

The following movements are just a sampling of what you and your spouse can do to interact with your baby. Check the Recommended Reading List (page 297) for other books on baby movements and exercises.

Pectoral Stretches

Benefits

- Stretches and strengthens pectoral muscles
- Releases tension in the shoulder area
- Tones all shoulder, elbow, forearm, wrist, and hand muscle groups
- Loosens and tones pectoralis muscle group and elbow flexors

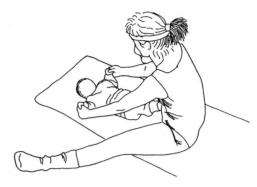

A. STRETCHING ARMS OPEN

Directions

1. Place your baby on his back. Have him clasp your thumbs, then wrap your fingers around his hands.
2. Gently stretch your baby's arms open (Figure 17.1A).
3. Cross both arms over his chest (Figure 17.1B).
4. Repeat 10 times.

Cautions and Comments

- Make the movements fun!
- Never force any movement. Tune into your baby and work with him.

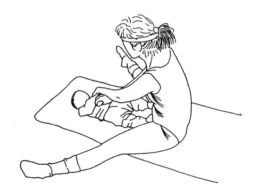

B. CROSSING HANDS OVER CHEST

Figure 17.1 Pectoral Stretches

Arm Stretches

Benefits

- Strengthens arms, shoulders, and chest
- Stretches contracted arm muscles
- Releases tension from shoulder area and arms
- Strengthens anterior chest and torso muscles (pectoralis muscle groups, latissimus dorsi, deltoids, trapezii)

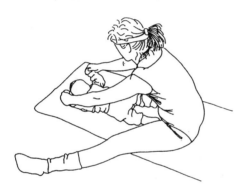

Figure 17.2 Arm Stretches

Directions

1. Place the baby on his back. Have him clasp your thumbs, then wrap your fingers around his hands.
2. Raise his arms straight above his head, then lower them to his sides (Figure 17.2).
3. Repeat 10 times.
4. Now, keeping his right arm at his side, raise his left arm over his head then bring it back down. Do this 10 times.
5. Repeat same movements using the other arm.

Cautions and Comments

- Keep the arm movements steady and smooth.
- Most babies tend to keep their arms bent during infancy. This movement helps stretch those contracted arm muscles.

Opposite Arm-to-Leg Stretch

Benefits

- Helps develop coordination
- Stretches posterior shoulder girdle, latissimus dorsi, thoraco-lumbar erector spinae, and gluteals

Directions

1. Place your baby on his back. Take his right hand in your left hand and his left foot in your right hand (Figure 17.3A).
2. Bring his foot and hand up until they meet above his body (Figure 17.3B).
3. Straighten his arm and leg before returning them to the starting position.
4. Repeat 10 times on each side.

Cautions and Comments

- This active movement can be useful in eliminating crankiness.
- Movements should be done slowly and with control.

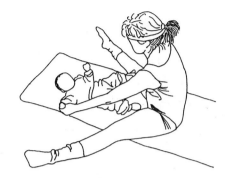

A. STARTING POSITION

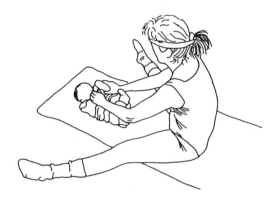

B. COMPLETED MOVEMENT

Figure 17.3 Opposite Arm-to-Leg Stretch

The Bicycle

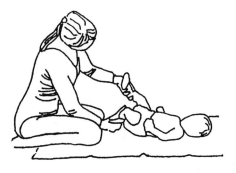

A. STARTING POSITION

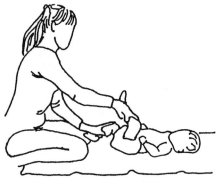

B. BICYCLING MOVEMENT

Figure 17.4   The Bicycle

Benefits

- Strengthens stomach muscles
- Keeps legs limber and supple
- Both strengthens and stretches ili-opsoas muscle group, gluteals and hip extensors, and rectus abdominalis

Directions

1. Place your baby on his back and grasp both of his legs in your hands (Figure 17.4A).
2. Rotate his legs as if he is riding a bicycle (Figure 17.4B).
3. Do 5-10 rotations.
4. Reverse direction and complete another 5-10 rotations.

Cautions and Comments

- Make your movements steady and not too fast.
- Most babies love this movement.

Leg Over Stretch

Benefits

- Releases tension from legs
- Stretches and tones thoraco-lumbar erector spinae, iliopsoas muscle group, hip adductors, gluteals, tensor fascia latae, and oblique abdominalis muscles

Directions

1. Place your baby on his back and hold his ankles (Figure 17.5A).
2. Gently move one leg over to the opposite side (Figure 17.5B), then return it to starting position.
3. Repeat 5-10 times with each leg.

Cautions and Comments

- Do not force the leg over.
- Use gentle, slow, rhythmic movements when doing this stretch.

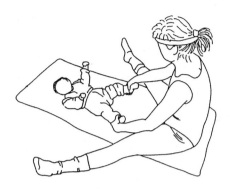

A. STARTING POSITION

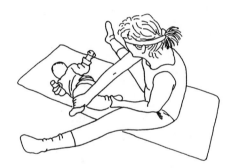

B. BRINGING LEG OVER

Figure 17.5 Leg Over Stretch

"V" Legs

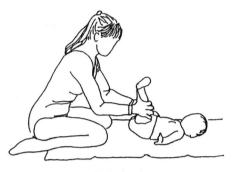

A. STARTING POSITION

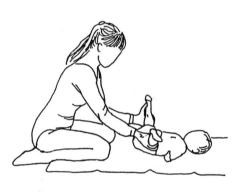

B. SEPARATING LEGS

Figure 17.6   "V" Legs

Benefits

- Strengthens stomach muscles
- Keeps legs strong and flexible
- Stretches and tones hip abductors and adductors, hip rotators, rectus abdominalis muscles, and knee extensors (quadriceps)

Directions

1. Place your baby on his back. Raise his legs and bring the soles of his feet together (Figure 17.6A).
2. Slowly separate his legs, lowering them carefully (Figure 17.6B).
3. Repeat 5-10 times.

Cautions and Comments

- *Do not force any movement!*
- Make sure you do not twist your baby's knees or pull his legs beyond a comfortable point.

Fanny Circles

Benefits

- Stretches legs and buttocks
- Stretches and strengthens lumbo-sacral erector spinae muscles, gluteals and hamstrings, and oblique abdominalis muscles

Directions

1. Place your baby on his back.
2. Hold both of his ankles in one hand and his buttocks in the other. Make a circular motion with his buttocks while keeping his legs fairly straight (Figure 17.7A).
3. Do 5-10 circles in both directions (Figure 17.7B).

Cautions and Comments

- Babies usually love this. Be prepared to hear laughter.
- Circle movements should be done slowly.

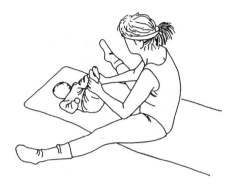

A. CIRCLING IN ONE DIRECTION...

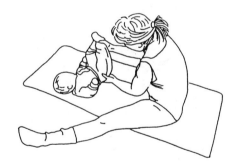

B. THEN THE OTHER

Figure 17.7 Fanny Circles

Toes-to-Nose Stretch

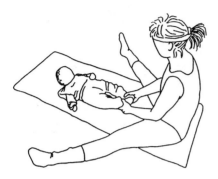

A. STARTING POSITION

- Tones abdominal muscles
- Increases flexibility in the legs and hips
- Stretches and tones the rectus and oblique abdominalis and iliopsoas muscle groups, gluteals, hamstrings, and thoraco-lumbar erector spinae

Directions

1. Place your baby on his back. Hold his feet and gently stretch his legs toward you (Figure 17.8A).
2. Gently fold his legs up toward his body, stretching his toes toward his nose (Figure 17.8B).
3. Repeat 5-10 times.

Cautions and Comments

- This movement is likely to delight your baby because his toes are often his favorite plaything.
- Use a smooth motion for this movement.

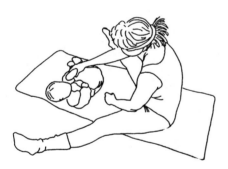

B. STRETCHING TOES TO NOSE

Figure 17.8 Toes-to-Nose Stretch

Froggy

Benefits

- Strengthens the leg muscles
- Strengthens and tones hip external rotators; hip abductors and adductors; iliopsoas muscle group; quadriceps; gluteals; cervical, thoracic, and lumbar erector spinae

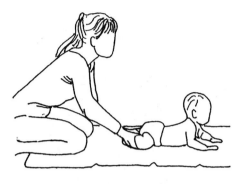

A. MOVING FEET UP

Directions

1. Place your baby on his tummy and hold his legs above the ankles.
2. Gently move his feet up toward his crotch, making sure to keep his legs on the blanket (Figure 17.9A).
3. Straighten both of his legs then spread them comfortably out to the sides (Figure 17.9B).
4. Bring his legs together making sure his knees are on the blanket (Figure 17.9C).
5. Repeat 5-10 times.

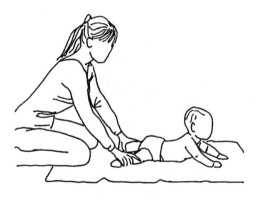

B. LEGS OUT TO SIDES

Cautions and Comments

- Though this exercise will not necessarily make your baby crawl at an early age, it will help him use the muscles needed for crawling.
- After several weeks of doing the Froggy, some babies begin to push themselves forward. This is a precrawling movement.

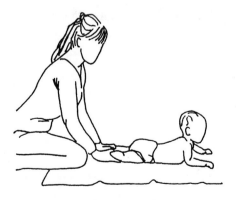

C. BRINGING KNEES TOGETHER

Figure 17.9   Froggy

Baby Sit-Ups

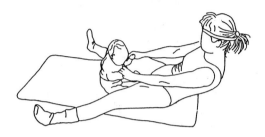

A. PULLING UP TO SITTING POSITION

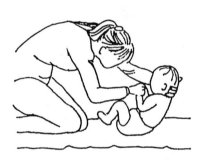

B. SUPPORTING BABY'S HEAD

Figure 17.10   Baby Sit-Ups

Benefits

- Stretches and strengthens the mom's abdominal muscles
- Tones cervical pre- and post-vertebral muscle groups, anterior shoulder/chest muscle groups, rectus abdominalis, and iliopsoas muscle group

Directions

1. Place your baby on his back between your outstretched legs. Let him grab your hand.
2. Slowly pull him up into a sitting position while you curl your back down closer to the mat (Figure 17.10A). If you baby is unable to hold his head up, place one of your hands behind his head for support (Figure 17.10B).
3. Slowly return to the starting position.
4. Repeat 5-10 times.

Cautions and Comments

- *Never let your baby's head fall backward!*
- Make sure you keep the movements slow.

Closing Thoughts
For New Parents

Early one morning many years ago, I was stretching in bed prior to getting up when I heard a rustling sound somewhere near my head. My older son, Mat, who was about six years old then and famous for leaving me notes, designs, pictures, and collages that he had made while waiting for me to get out of bed, had left something on my pillow. I looked over and found the following note:

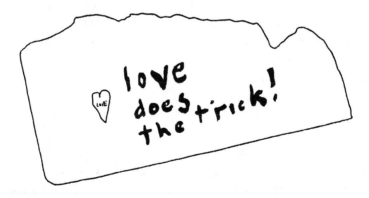

I was touched by his message and his understanding of how the world operates. How pleasant it was to receive a message like that from my own son. I put that special note in a safe place so that I could refer to it whenever my tolerance, patience, or sense of humor were waning.

To me, the note's message represents half of a balanced approach to parenting. The other half is maintaining consistent discipline. By blending love and discipline in a balanced way, you will find success and enjoyment in your parenting role.

YOUR CHILD IS A GIFT

It is wise to think of your child as a precious gift that you have been given to love, teach, discipline, and, most importantly, to enjoy. From the very beginning, even when your baby was growing inside of you, you should have realized that he or she was a unique individual and should be respected as such.

Your child will have many things to share with you as he grows. I am continually amazed by the varied interests that my children pursue. In many cases, they are interested in topics that I have never even wondered about. Sharing their interests has broadened my horizons, and it has increased their faith in themselves and in their abilities. In return, I have taught them such things as deep, slow breathing for those nights when sleep won't come.

My children are older now—in college, in fact—but our attitude of mutual respect and sharing has always been there from the beginning. The easiest way to accomplish this is through open and continual communication. The more you explain your feelings, the deeper the relationship and respect you will share with your children. Tell them your reasons for doing certain things and not doing others. Start by talking to your child when he is in utero. Tell him how you feel while he is growing inside of you. Continue open communication after your baby is born; eventually he will come to understand your words. Even before your child has developed language skills, he will still benefit from your gestures, facial expressions, and the sound of your voice.

As your child grows and is able to verbalize his own feelings, take time to listen. Look directly at your child and maintain constant eye contact as he tells you all about the hurt, frustration, or joy of the moment. Taking time (sometimes it's only twenty seconds) to concentrate on and respect what your child has to say, helps in developing his self-respect as well as a loving parent-child relationship.

PARENT OR FRIEND?

Many parents fall into the trap of trading their parental role, which requires both love and discipline, for the role of a friend, which requires only love. The parent who chooses to eliminate the more consistent and responsible aspects of parenting is essentially rejecting the more difficult aspects of this role. If you choose to do a good job in your role as parent, it is important that you assume responsibility for *all* the jobs that the role demands.

One of the easiest ways to fulfill the disciplinary aspect of parenting is to increase your own self-discipline so you set a good example for your child. Obviously, a daily exercise program with your child will fulfill this need. As your baby grows, he will participate more and more in these practice sessions. Talk to, hug, and kiss your baby as you practice. Mix love for your baby with a program of self-love and self-discipline. You will welcome the results!

ACCENTUATE THE POSITIVE

As you and your child grow, condition yourself to turn negative thoughts and behavior into positive ones. This concept can easily apply to a program of behavior modification. Learn to recognize the positive aspects of what your child says, does, and creates while playing down the negative aspects. This doesn't mean that when your child has done something that violates the rules of the household that he should go unpunished. What it does mean, rather, is that you should continually build your child's self-respect by noticing all the positive things he does. This is easier to do when you are not on a hectic schedule; often when things get harried, positive statements can easily get lost. Try to train yourself to notice at least one positive thing about yourself and your child each day. Taking the extra few minutes to think about and express these ideas can have very beneficial results. It makes it easier for you to enjoy the parental role while improving your child's development.

HAVE FUN WITH YOUR CHILD

Having a sense of humor and not taking your parenting role too seriously can work wonders! You may find that your child teaches you about life. By blending humor, love, discipline, and patience into the pattern of your daily life, you can have fun. Don't worry about doing everything perfectly. Let the love you feel for your mate and your child radiate for all the world to see. Remember the simple truth my son taught me: love does the trick!

Appendices

Glossary

Abdominal breath. A deep breath experienced by inhaling and moving the lower abdomen forward and exhaling by contracting the lower abdominal area. Will calm and revitalize the body and mind.

Affirmations. Prayer, self suggestions for a positive purpose. A constant thought of what you want.

Afterpains. The uterine cramps due to contracting efforts of the uterus to return to normal size. Occurs during the first few days after birth. Afterpains may be more severe during breastfeeding and with subsequent children.

Allopathy. Rational, scientific and conventional medicine.

Amino Acids. The building blocks of protein; twenty different amino acids are commonly found in protein.

Anal muscles. Muscles that open and close the rectal outlet.

Anemia. A condition in which the red corpuscles of the blood are reduced in number or are deficient in hemoglobin.

Anus. Muscular outlet of the rectum, which is the lower end of the large intestine.

Areola. The brown area surrounding the nipples; its function is protecting the nipples during nursing.

Awareness. Consciousness; open attention or being in the here and now.

Birth canal. The cavity of the uterus and vagina through which the baby passes at birth.

Bleeding. Menstruation; when excessive, called hemorrhage.

Breastfeeding. Nourishing your baby with the milk produced in your breasts.

Calmative technique. Any technique that

has a calming effect on your body. Massage and calming music as well as herbal teas are examples.

Colic. The painful stomach or intestinal spasms sometimes suffered by new babies, usually during the first three months of life.

Colostrum. The first fluid secreted by the mother's breasts before her milk arrives. It is high in antibodies and protein, which protect the nursing baby from possible infections and allergies.

Contraction. A tensing or shortening of the muscle fibers of the uterus, which is followed by a relaxation or lengthening of these fibers.

Diaphragm. A large, thick muscle that separates the chest (thorax) from the abdomen. This is the muscle used in the "Abdominal Breath."

Engorged breasts. Milk-laden breasts from which the milk is not flowing.

Episiotomy. A surgical incision or cut (usually made with scissors) of the perineum (outer birth canal) to give the baby's head more room, to prevent tearing of the vagina, and to make the birth smoother.

Expressing milk. The process of extracting milk from the breasts to be used at a later feeding or to relieve engorged breasts. Milk can be expressed by using one's hand or by means of a breast pump.

Hemorrhoids. Inflamed and often painful veins of the rectum.

Herbs. Any of a variety of often aromatic plants that are used especially in medicine.

Hindmilk. The breast milk released in the last part of the feeding; it has the highest fat content.

Hormone. From the Greek word meaning "to stimulate," hormones are substances that are produced in one part of the body and specifically influence certain activities of cells in other parts of the body.

Lactation. The secretion or formation of milk, or the period of milk production in the female body.

Let-down reflex. The baby's sucking stimulates the mother's pituitary gland (located at the base of the brain) to secrete oxytocin. During each nursing, this causes the milk sacs to tighten and squeeze milk down to the milk-collecting sinuses. May be felt by the mother as a squeezing or tingling in the breast or may be undetectable.

Lochia. Vaginal discharge made up of blood, mucus, and tissue from the uterus and vagina after delivery. May last four to eight weeks.

Mastitis. Inflammation of the breast; it may be accompanied with a breast abscess.

Meditation. The relaxation of the body and the quieting of the mind during concentration on the breath, or an internal or external sound.

Midwife. A person who assists women in childbirth.

Multigravida. A woman who has been pregnant more than once.

Multipara. A woman who has borne more

than one child. Also called multip.

Oxytocin. A hormone produced by the pituitary gland that stimulates uterine contractions and the let-down reflex. Nipple stimulation during breastfeeding causes the release of oxytocin.

Pelvic floor. Muscle layers that form a sling across the base of the pelvis and support the bladder, uterus, and rectum.

Pelvis. The bones that form the two hip bones: the sacrum and the tailbone. Contain the regenerative organs of the female.

Piles. Another term for hemorrhoids.

Postpartum. The period of time following the birth of the baby, before the mother returns to her prepregnancy condition.

Prenatal. The time period during pregnancy before the baby is born.

Primipara. A woman who has given birth to her first child. Also called primip.

Rooting instinct. Natural movement of the baby's head toward the cheek that is touched or stroked.

Round ligaments. Fibrous muscles connecting the uterus and the pelvic bones.

Stress. A mental or physical strain, urgency, or pressure.

Tofu. Soaked, cooked, and curdled soybeans used in Asian cooking. It is high in quality proteins and low in fat.

Urethra. The narrow passageway through which urine is discharged from the bladder.

Uterus. The womb in which the baby develops during the nine months of pregnancy.

Vagina. The muscular birth canal leading from the uterus to the outer genitals.

Varicose veins. Swollen, painful veins, usually of the legs but often found in the genitals as well.

Water-soluble vitamins. Found in the water portion of foods, these substances are needed in small quantities for health and well-being. B-complex vitamins and Vitamin C are examples.

Weaning. The gradual withholding of breast milk from your baby when the introduction of solid food begins.

Muscles of the Human Body

Front — Complete Musculature

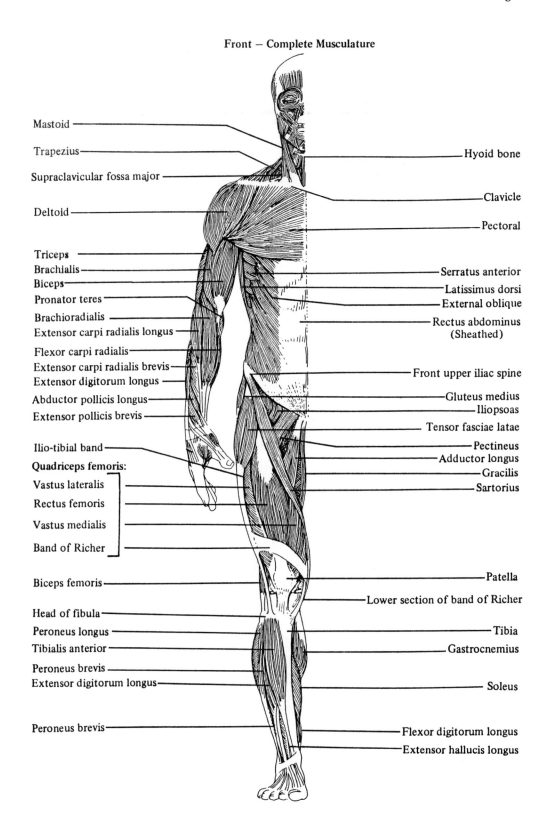

Mastoid

Trapezius

Supraclavicular fossa major

Deltoid

Triceps
Brachialis
Biceps
Pronator teres
Brachioradialis
Extensor carpi radialis longus
Flexor carpi radialis
Extensor carpi radialis brevis
Extensor digitorum longus
Abductor pollicis longus
Extensor pollicis brevis

Ilio-tibial band
Quadriceps femoris:
Vastus lateralis
Rectus femoris
Vastus medialis
Band of Richer

Biceps femoris

Head of fibula
Peroneus longus
Tibialis anterior
Peroneus brevis
Extensor digitorum longus

Peroneus brevis

Hyoid bone

Clavicle

Pectoral

Serratus anterior
Latissimus dorsi
External oblique
Rectus abdominus
(Sheathed)

Front upper iliac spine
Gluteus medius
Iliopsoas
Tensor fasciae latae
Pectineus
Adductor longus
Gracilis
Sartorius

Patella
Lower section of band of Richer

Tibia
Gastrocnemius

Soleus

Flexor digitorum longus
Extensor hallucis longus

Back — Complete Musculature

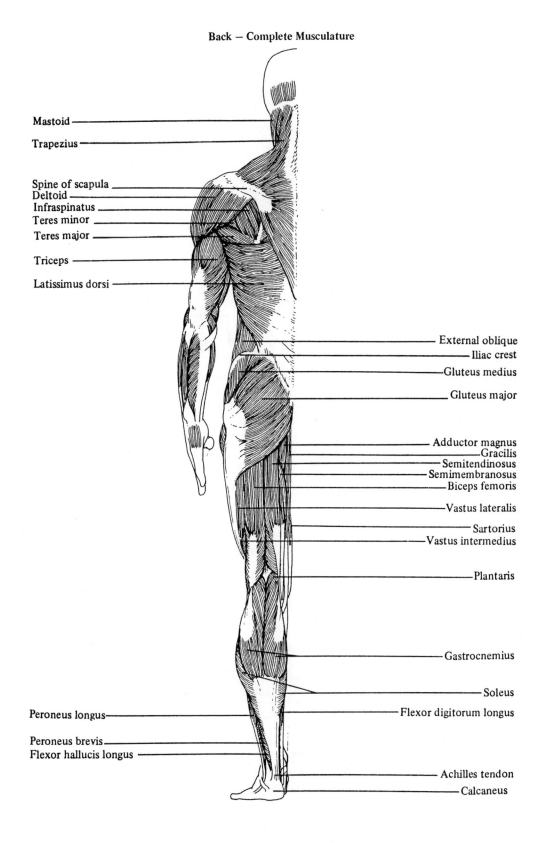

Mastoid

Trapezius

Spine of scapula
Deltoid
Infraspinatus
Teres minor
Teres major

Triceps

Latissimus dorsi

External oblique
Iliac crest
Gluteus medius

Gluteus major

Adductor magnus
Gracilis
Semitendinosus
Semimembranosus
Biceps femoris

Vastus lateralis

Sartorius
Vastus intermedius

Plantaris

Gastrocnemius

Soleus

Peroneus longus

Flexor digitorum longus

Peroneus brevis
Flexor hallucis longus

Achilles tendon
Calcaneus

Side — Full Musculature

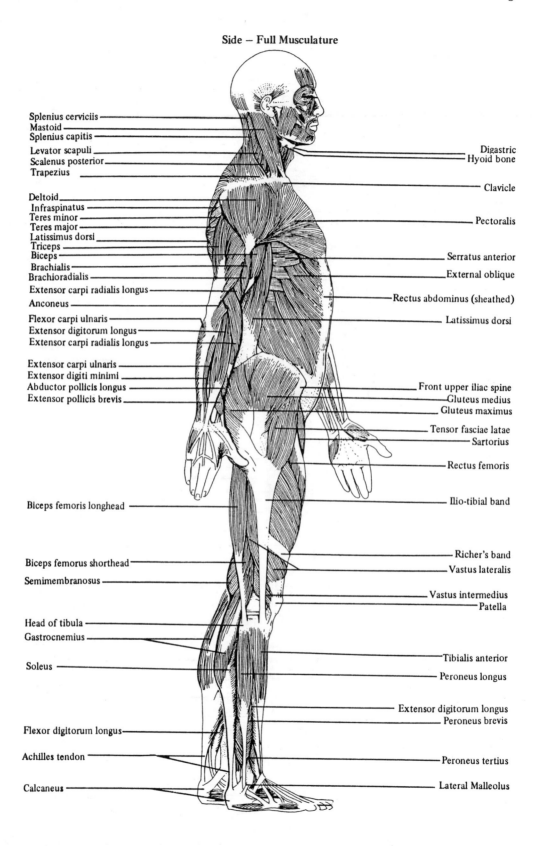

Splenius cerviciis
Mastoid
Splenius capitis
Levator scapuli
Scalenus posterior
Trapezius

Deltoid
Infraspinatus
Teres minor
Teres major
Latissimus dorsi
Triceps
Biceps
Brachialis
Brachioradialis
Extensor carpi radialis longus
Anconeus
Flexor carpi ulnaris
Extensor digitorum longus
Extensor carpi radialis longus

Extensor carpi ulnaris
Extensor digiti minimi
Abductor pollicis longus
Extensor pollicis brevis

Biceps femoris longhead

Biceps femorus shorthead
Semimembranosus

Head of tibula
Gastrocnemius

Soleus

Flexor digitorum longus

Achilles tendon

Calcaneus

Digastric
Hyoid bone

Clavicle

Pectoralis

Serratus anterior
External oblique

Rectus abdominus (sheathed)

Latissimus dorsi

Front upper iliac spine
Gluteus medius
Gluteus maximus

Tensor fasciae latae
Sartorius

Rectus femoris

Ilio-tibial band

Richer's band
Vastus lateralis

Vastus intermedius
Patella

Tibialis anterior
Peroneus longus

Extensor digitorum longus
Peroneus brevis

Peroneus tertius

Lateral Malleolus

Recommended Reading and Viewing

Unless otherwise indicated, the following books can be ordered from:

Birth and Life Bookstore
7001 Alonzo Avenue NW
PO Box 70625
Seattle, WA 98107-0625

(800) 736-0631
(206) 789-4444

BREASTFEEDING

Dana, Nancy, and Anne Price. *Working Woman's Guide to Breastfeeding.* Rev. ed. Minneapolis, MN: Meadowbrook Press, 1987.

Addresses the special needs of breastfeeding mothers who work outside the home.

Huggins, Kathleen. *The Nursing Mother's Companion.* Boston, MA: Harvard Common Press, 1986.

A lucid, trouble-shooting aid for the new mother who is learning how to nurse.

Kitzinger, Sheila. *Breastfeeding Your Baby.* New York: Alfred A. Knopf, 1989.

A reassuring breastfeeding guide with outstanding photos and illustrations, many in color.

La Leche League, International. *The Womanly Art of Breastfeeding.* 4th ed. Franklin Park, IL: La Leche League, International, 1987.

A practical manual of "good mothering through breastfeeding" by the acknowledged experts.

Woessner, Candace, Judith Lauwers, and Barbara Bernard. *Breastfeeding Today, A Mother's Companion.* 2d ed. Garden City Park, NY: Avery Publishing Group, 1991.

Practical advice and up-to-date information on breastfeeding by the authors of Counseling the Nursing Mother.

CESAREAN BIRTH

Ancheta, Ruth. *VBAC Book: Vaginal Birth After Cesarean.* Elm Grove, WI: Birth Information, 1987.

Overview of vaginal birth after Cesarean delivery for professionals and parents.

Cohen, Nancy Wainer. *Open Season!* Westport, CT: Greenwood Press, 1991.

A healing update of the alarming number of Cesarean births and the growing popularity and acceptance of vaginal birth after Cesarean delivery. (Order through Be Healthy, Inc., *page 307.)*

Cohen, Nancy Wainer, and Lois Estner. *Silent Knife: Cesarean Prevention and Vaginal Birth After Cesarean.* Granby, MA: Bergin & Garvey Publishers, 1983.

Powerful, impassioned, thoroughly documented critique of the growing reliance on Cesarean births. Includes strategies to prevent unnecessary Cesarean deliveries. (Order through Be Healthy, Inc., *page 307.)*

Richards, Lynn Baptisti, et al. *The Vaginal Birth After Cesarean Experience.* Granby, MA: Bergin & Garvey Publishers, 1987.

Covers a wide range of birthing issues through birth stories by parents and professionals.

CHILD CARE

Bettelheim, Bruno. *A Good Enough Parent: A Book on Child-Rearing.* New York: Alfred A. Knopf, 1987.

Deals with misconceptions on being a "perfect" parent.

Brazelton, T. Berry. *Toddlers and Parents, A Declaration of Independence.* Rev. ed. New York: Delta Books, 1989.

How to survive and enjoy your one-, two-, or three-year old.

Briggs, Dorothy Corkille. *Your Child's Self-Esteem.* Garden City, NY: Doubleday, 1975.

How to create feelings of self-worth, your child's most important characteristic.

Crary, Elizabeth. *Without Spanking or Spoiling.* Seattle, WA: Parenting Press, 1979.

Alternatives for parents in attaining their personal goals in child rearing.

Dinkmeyer, Don, and Gary McKay. The *Parent's Handbook: Systematic Training for Effective Parenting (STEP).* Rev. ed. Circle Pines, MN: American Guidance Service, 1989.

STEP program handbook for effective communication and discipline by natural consequences.

Dodson, Fitzhugh. *How to Discipline—With Love.* New York: New American Library, 1977.

Strategies when disciplining children from the crib stage to college age.

Driscoll, Jeanne, and Marsha Walker. *Taking Care of Your New Baby.* Garden City Park, NY: Avery Publishing Group, 1989.

A comprehensive guide to infant care.

Eisenberg, Arlene, Heidi Eisenberg Markoff, and Sandee Eisenberg Hathaway. *What to Expect the First Year.* New York: Workman Publishing Co., 1989.

Readable, reassuring, comprehensive, month-by-month guide of everything parents need to know during their child's first year.

Fraiberg, Selma. *The Magic Years: Understanding and Handling the Problems of Early Childhood.* New York: Charles Scribner's Sons, 1959.

Insight into the inner life of a young child. A classic. Highly recommended.

Glenn, H. Stephen, and Jane Nelson. *Raising Self-Reliant Children in a Self-Indulgent World.* New York: Prima Publishing, 1989.

Strategies for developing capable young people.

Leach, Penelope. *Your Baby & Child, From Birth to Age Five.* Rev. ed. New York: Alfred A. Knopf, 1989.

Comprehensive, sensitive guide to child care and development. Beautifully illustrated.

Sears, William. *Creative Parenting.* Rev. ed. New York: Dodd, Mead & Company, 1987.

Discusses the concept of "attachment parenting" in the successful raising of children from birth to adolescence.

White, Burton. *The First Three Years of Life.* Rev. ed. Englewood Cliffs, NJ: Prentice-Hall, 1985.

Detailed guide on the development of the young child.

CHILD CARE VIDEO

Your Baby: A Video Guide to Care and Understanding with Penelope Leach.

Comprehensive and practical guide to newborn baby care and development. Penelope Leach, noted best-selling author of Your Baby and Child and mother of two children, demonstrates techniques of everyday care and teaches you exactly what your baby needs from you. (Order through Be Healthy, Inc., *page 307.)*

COOKBOOKS

Johnson, Roberta. *Whole Foods for the Whole Family.* New York: New American Library, 1981.

The La Leche League cookbook. This book is a basic introduction to improving a family's nutrition with healthy, delicious recipes.

Katzen, Mollie. *Moosewood Cookbook.* Berkeley, CA: Ten Speed Press, 1977.

A beautifully illustrated, creative vegetarian cookbook. Tasty and inventive recipes. Highly recommended.

Katzen, Mollie. *The Enchanted Broccoli Forest.* Berkeley, CA: Ten Speed Press, 1982.

More creative, tasty recipes from Mollie. Includes a chapter on bread baking. Highly recommended.

Lappé, Frances Moore. *Diet for a Small Planet.* Rev. ed. New York: Bantam Books, 1984.

The source book on complementary proteins. An excellent discussion on how incomplete proteins can be combined to produce high-grade protein nutrition. Also contains a variety of recipes to put these ideas into practice.

Robertson, Laurel. *New Laurel's Kitchen.* Rev. ed. Berkeley, CA: Ten Speed Press, 1986.

Classic vegetarian, natural foods cookbook and reference. Completely revised.

Satter, Ellyn. *Child of Mine: Feeding with Love and Good Sense.* Rev. ed. Palo Alto, CA: Bull Publishing, 1986.

Common-sense guide for parents based on nutritional science and human relationships.

DEPRESSION (POSTPARTUM)

Dalton, Katherine. *Depression After Childbirth.* New York: Oxford University Press, 1989.

Excellent publication dealing with postpartum depression.

Dix, Carol. *The New Mother Syndrome: Coping with Postpartum Stress and Depression.* New York: Pocket Books, 1988.

Useful book for coping with postpartum depression. Available through DAD (Depression After Delivery) National, PO Box 1282, Morrisville, PA 19067. (215) 295-3994.

Greun, Dawn. *The New Parent: A Spectrum of Postpartum Adjustment.* Seattle, WA: Pennypress, 1988.

Fine discussion of postpartum life as well as depression. Send $1.00 to Pennypress, Inc., 1100 23rd Avenue East, Seattle, WA 98112. (206) 325-1419.

Pacific Postpartum Support Society. *Postpartum Depression and Anxiety: A Self-Help Guide for Mothers.*

Helpful guide for postpartum depression and the blues. Available through Pacific Postpartum Support Society, 1416 Commercial Drive, Suite 104, Vancouver, BC, Canada V5L 3X9. (604) 255-7999.

EXERCISES

Feinup-Riordan, Ann. *Shape Up with Baby: Exercise Games for the New Parent and Child.* Seattle, WA: Pennypress, 1980.

Exercises that are fun for both mother and baby.

Levy, Janine. *The Baby Exercise Book.* New York: Pantheon Press, 1975.

Detailed exercises for the first fifteen months of life.

Noble, Elizabeth. *Marie Osmond's Exercises for Mothers and Babies.* Harrisonburg, VA: New American Library, 1985.

Gentle, effective postpartum exercises and baby movements. (Order through Be Healthy, Inc., page 307.)

O'Brien, Paddy. *Your Life After Birth: Exercises and Meditations for the First Year of Motherhood.* Boston, MA: Pandora, 1988.

Practical handbook draws on women's per-

sonal accounts of postpartum feelings and experiences.

Regnier, Susan L. *You and Me, Baby: A Prenatal, Postpartum, Infant Exercise Book.* Deephaven, MN: Meadowbrook Press, 1984.

The YMCA's program for prenatal and postpartum fitness.

Walker, Peter, and Fiona Walker. *Natural Parenting, A Practical Guide for Fathers and Mothers: Conception to Age Three.* Brooklyn, NY: Interlink Publishing Group, 1987.

A baby and parent workout book with exercise and massage programs formulated by an experienced yoga and exercise teacher who specializes in working with babies.

Whiteford, Barbara, and Margie Polden. *The Postnatal Exercise Book.* New York: Pantheon Press, 1984.

An innovative postpartum exercise program developed in England. Includes water exercises.

EXERCISE VIDEOS

The following videos are recommended to be used in conjunction with this book. They are available through:

Collage Video Specialties, Inc.
5390 Main Street NE, Dept. 1
Minneapolis, MN 55421
(800) 433-6769
(612) 571-5840

Austin, Denise. *Stretch and Flex.* Newark, NJ: Parade Video, 1989.

Soothing, new-age music in a mellow work-

out by noted fitness expert Denise Austin. *Extremely relaxing stretches. 30 minutes.*

Fonda, Jane. *Low-Impact Aerobics.* Burbank, CA: Warner Home Video, 1986.

Jane Fonda's only pure low-impact aerobics tape. Great for beginning and intermediate exercisers. Fun tape to work with. 53 minutes.

Prudden, Suzy. *Meta-Fitness: A Unique Body/ Mind Workout Video.* Santa Monica, CA: Hay House, Inc., 1989.

Multidimensional approach includes invigorating exercises with Bonnie Prudden as well as positive affirmations for your subconscious by Louise Hay. Excellent relaxation exercises included. All stomach-flattening exercises in this book are found on this video. 59 minutes.

Simmons, Richard. *Sweatin' to the Oldies.* Burbank, CA: Warner Home Video, 1988.

An aerobic concert with Richard Simmons featuring songs of the sixties plus easy-to-follow movements. Fun tape to work with. 58 minutes.

FATHERING

Sears, William. *Becoming a Father.* Franklin Park, IL: La Leche League, International, 1986.

The joys and problems of parenthood from the male perspective. Highly recommended. (Order through Be Healthy, Inc., page 307.)

Shapiro, Jerrold Lee. *When Men are Pregnant: Needs and Concerns of Expectant Fathers.* Saint Luis Obispo, CA: Impact

Publishers, 1987.

This book helps expectant fathers make sense of the earliest experiences of fatherhood. Highly recommended.

Syndal, Larry, and Carl Jones. *The New Father Survival Guide.* New York: Franklin Watts Inc., 1987.

A light-hearted and sympathetic aid for coping with the early days of fatherhood.

HEALTH CARE (CHILDREN'S)

Jones, Sandy. *Guide to Baby Products.* Rev. ed. New York: Consumer Reports Books, 1989.

Baby products with an emphasis on safety and convenience.

Samuels, Mike, and Nancy Samuels. *The Well Baby Book.* New York: Summit Books, 1979.

Holistic approach to pregnancy and child care.

Spock, Benjamin, MD, and Michael Rothenberg, MD. *Dr. Spock's Baby and Child Care.* Rev. ed. New York: Simon and Schuster, 1985.

The revised classic source book for parents.

Stoppard, Miriam. *Baby and Child A to Z Medical Handbook.* Los Angeles, CA: The Body Press, 1986.

Reference to help parents respond to their children's common medical problems.

HERBS

Parvati, Jeannine. *HYGIEIA: A Woman's Herbal.* Monroe, UT: Freestone Collective Books, 1978.

Interweaves ancient herbal practices and techniques with new women's consciousness and holistic health. (Order through Be Healthy, Inc., page 307.)

Weed, Susun S. *Wise Woman Herbal for the Childbearing Year.* Woodstock, NY: Ash Tree Publishing, 1987.

Comprehensive guide for everyone involved in women's health. Gives detailed instructions for herbal usage during pregnancy and the postpartum period. (Order through Be Healthy, Inc., page 307.)

MASSAGE (INFANT)

Auckett, Amelia, *Baby Massage: Parent-Child Bonding Through Touching.* Rev. ed. New York: Newmarket Press, 1989.

Techniques and health benefits of caring touch.

Leboyer, Frederick. *Loving Hands.* New York: Random House, 1976.

The traditional Indian art of baby massage.

Montagu, Ashley. *Touching: The Human Significance of the Skin.* 3d ed. New York: Harper & Row Publishers, 1986.

Tactile experience is as important as breathing, eating, or resting to the survival of humans.

McClure, Vimala Schneider. *Infant Massage: A Handbook for Loving Parents.* Rev. ed. New York: Bantam Books, 1989.

Massage program to enhance infant development. (Order through Be Healthy, Inc., page 307)

Ohashi, Wataru, and Mary Stewart. *Touch for Love: Shiatsu for Your Baby.* New York: Ballantine Books, 1985.

Acupressure for babies.

Walker, Peter. *The Book of Baby Massage: For a Happier, Healthier Child.* New York: Simon & Schuster, 1988.

Contains a series of gentle, playful massage sequences designed to open up a relaxed physical dialogue between parents and baby.

MASSAGE (PARENTS)

Bauer, Cathryn. *Acupressure for Women.* Freedom, CA: Crossing Press, 1987.

Simple finger pressure can be a safe and effective alternative to drug therapy for PMS, menstrual cramps, stress, painful labor contractions, and menopausal hot flashes.

Byers, Dwight. *Better Health with Foot Reflexology.* Florida: Ingham Publishing Company, 1983.

Detailed explanation and technique for foot reflexology.

Downing, George. *The Massage Book.* Rev. ed. New York: Random House, 1981.

Good basic massage book featuring Swedish massage techniques. Contains detailed illustrations.

Hudson, Clare Maxwell. *The Complete Book of Massage.* New York: Random House, 1988.

Detailed and complete book explaining total massage.

Lidell, Lucina. *The Book of Massage: The Complete Step-by-Step Guide to Eastern and Western Techniques.* New York: Simon & Schuster, 1984.

Shiatsu (acupressure) and foot reflexology are included in this complete guide.

Ohashi, Wataru. *Do It Yourself Shiatsu: How to Perform the Ancient Japanese Art of Acupuncture without Needles.* New York: E.P. Dutton, 1976.

Thorough, detailed book on shiatsu massage therapy.

Tappen, Frances M. *Healing Massage Techniques: A Study of Eastern and Western Methods.* Reston, VA: Reston Publishing Co., 1978.

Discusses various methods of body work.

NUTRITION

Baker, Susan, and Roberta Henry. *Parent's Guide to Nutrition: Healthy Eating from Birth through Adolescence.* Reading, MA: Addison-Wesley, 1986.

From Boston Children's Hospital, this book contains comprehensive information on the principles of nutrition for children.

Erick, Miriam. *D.I.E.T. During Pregnancy: The Complete Guide and Calendar.* Brookline, MA: Grinnen-Barret, 1987.

Calendar covers the weeks of pregnancy and one year of your baby's growth. Also contains helpful postpartum information as well as delicious, healthful recipes. (Order through Be Healthy, Inc., *page 307.)*

Kamen, Betty, PhD, and Si Kamen. *Total Nutrition for Breastfeeding Mothers.* Boston, MA: Little, Brown & Co., 1986.

Tells nursing mothers how to change their diet to improve the quality of their milk.

PARENTING

Bradshaw, John. *Bradshaw on The Family: A Revolutionary Way of Self-Discovery.* Deerfield Beach, FL: Health Communications, 1988.

The impact of family on personality formation. Included is helpful information on breaking the negative rules that have been formed as the result of dysfunctional family life.

Clarke, Jean Illsley. *Growing Up Again: Parenting Ourselves, Parenting Our Children.* San Francisco, CA: Winston, 1989.

Provides a total model for parenting.

Galinsky, Ellen. *The Six Stages of Parenthood.* Rev. ed. Reading, MA: Addison-Wesley Publishing Co., 1987.

Griffith, Linda Lewis. *Battle Fatigue...And You Thought You Were Busy Before You Had Children.* San Luis Obispo, CA: Impact Publishers, 1986.

Perspective, insight, and good humor to help mothers cope while taking care of themselves and their families.

Holt, Pat, and Grace Ketterman. *When You Feel Like Screaming! Help for Frustrated Mothers.* Wheaton, IL: Harold Shaw Publishers, 1988.

Explains why mothers scream, how it affects their kids, and how to achieve quiet control of self and family.

Lansky, Vicki. *Practical Parenting Tips.* Deephaven, MN: Meadowbrook, 1980.

The most practical guide for new parents. Over 1,000 super ideas to make parenting easier. (Order through Be Healthy, Inc., *page 307.)*

Satir, Virginia. *The New Peoplemaking.* Rev. ed. Palo Alto, CA: Science and Behavior Books, 1988.

Family life: its health and survival.

PLAYING AND LEARNING

Martin, Elaine. *Baby Games.* Philadelphia, PA: Running Press, 1988.

Suggests hundreds of rhymes, songs, finger plays, and games to entertain children from infancy through pre-school.

Munger, Evelyn Moats, and Susan Jane Bowdon. *The New Beyond Peek-a-Boo and*

Pat-a-Cake Activities for Baby's First Eighteen Months. Piscataway, NJ: New Century Publishers, 1986.

Games, songs, exercises, developmental and health information, and strategies for parents.

Shea, Jan Fisher. *No Bored Babies*. Seattle, WA: Bear Creek Publications, 1986.

Simple, inexpensive, and safe developmental toys for newborns and babies up to age two.

RELAXATION

Benson, Herbert. *The Relaxation Response.* Rev. ed. New York: Avon Books, 1982.

The classic book on relaxation and the use of meditation to achieve it.

Nuernberger, Phil, PhD. *Freedom from Stress: A Holistic Approach.* Honesdale, PA: Himalayan International, 1985.

Unique blend of science, common sense, and exercise in this practical approach to stress management.

Levey, Joel, PhD, and Michelle Levey. *The Fine Art of Relaxation, Concentration and Meditation.* London: Wisdom Publications, 1987.

Dr. Joel Levey leads the reader from simple self-regulation to self-knowledge and spiritual awareness. Available through Humankind, 5536 Woodlawn Avenue North, Seattle, WA 98103.

Zemach-Bersin, Davis, Kaethe Zamach-Bersin, and Mark Reese. *Relaxercise.* New

York: Harper & Row Publishers, 1990.

How to reprogram your neuromuscular system to stop pain and reduce stress. Based on the work of Moshe Feldenkrais. Novel approach to stress-related problems.

SEXUALITY

Bing, Elizabeth, and Libby Coleman. *Making Love During Pregnancy.* New York: Random House, 1990.

Thoroughly explains the sexual conflicts and emotions during pregnancy and postpartum. Highly recommended.

Kitzinger, Sheila. *Sex After the Baby Comes.* Seattle, WA: Pennypress, 1986.

An understanding look at resuming sex after giving birth.

———. *Women's Experiences of Sex.* New York: Alfred A. Knopf, 1983.

Explores all the sexual stages in a woman's life.

Zilbergeld, S. *Male Sexuality.* New York: St. Martin's Press, 1981.

Deals with the physical and emotional aspects of sex, discarding stereotypes and myths.

YOGA AND MEDITATION

Folan, Lilias. *Lilias, Yoga and Your Life.* New York: Macmillan Publishing Co., 1982.

A well-illustrated guide to beginning hatha yoga by Lilias, a leading teacher in the field.

Peck, Robert. *American Meditation and Beginning Yoga.* Lebanon, CT: Personal Development Center, 1976.

A clear, concise scientific exploration of yoga and meditation including chapters on left and right brain functions, deep-breathing exercises, altered states of consciousness, yoga philosophy, sensory and pain control, and kundalini yoga. Available through B. Peck, 67 Bush Hill Road, Lebanon, CT 06249.

Staff of the Kripalu Center. *The Self-Health Guide.* Lenox, MA: Kripalu Shop, 1983.

An excellent introduction to yoga and how the use of different techniques can help you achieve a radiant state of well-being. Write to: Kripalu Shop, Box 774, Dept. M, Lenox, MA 01240.

YOGA VIDEOS

Folan, Lilias. *Lilias! Yoga Videos.* Volume I: Beginners; Volume II: Intermediates. Cambridge, MA: Rudra Press, 1988.

Lilias has been on PBS for years. She is warm, enthusiastic, and exceptionally knowledgeable about yoga. Available through Rudra Press, PO Box 1973, Cambridge, MA, 02238. (800) 876-7798.

Yoga Journal. *Yoga for Beginners* with Patricia Walden. Santa Monica, CA: Healing Arts Home Video.

Presents a wide range of yoga postures and relaxation techniques. Helps you create your own personal program. Also includes a 48-page yoga handbook. Available through Healing Arts Home Video, 1229 Third Street, Santa Monica, CA, 90401. (800) 722-7347.

Mail-Order Products

Positive Parenting and Parenting Fitness tapes, books, and products are available to you through our mail-order company, *Be Healthy, Inc.* To order any of the products below, call or write:

Be Healthy, Inc.
51 Salt Rock Road
Baltic, CT 06330
(800) 433-5523   (203) 822-8573

We accept Mastercard and Visa. All orders are shipped UPS, so please remember to include your street address along with $3.50 for shipping and handling. All orders are shipped within five working days. Also, please keep in mind that prices are subject to change.

The products listed below are just a sampling of the over 80 items that *Be Healthy, Inc.* carries. For a complete 20-page catalog, send $2.00 to the above address. You will receive the catalog plus a $5.00 coupon to be used toward your purchase.

Positive Pregnancy and Parenting Fitness is a national organization that trains instructors to teach pregnancy and parenting fitness programs. For your $25.00 Parent Support Membership Fee, you will receive a 10 percent membership discount on all the items offered in the *Be Healthy* catalog, a copy of our biannual newsletter, and discounts on our workshops, which are offered throughout the United States.

Our newsletters contain articles on pregnancy and parenting that are designed to stimulate and enlighten. These newsletters contain book reviews, audio- and video-tape reviews, recipes, and lots of practical information for new parents and soon-to-be parents.

We sponsor Positive Pregnancy and Parenting Fitness Teacher-Training Workshops across the country. These workshops are listed on the Calendar of Events found in our newsletter. As a member, you will receive a substantial membership discount if you want to be trained to teach our programs.

I personally urge you to join our vital organization and take advantage of all it has to offer! If you are already a member, please include your current membership number with your order.

If you have any personal inquiries, feel free to write to me, Sylvia Klein Olkin, at the above address. I'd be happy to hear from you.

BOOKS

Becoming a Father: How to Nurture and Enjoy Your Family (La Leche League, 1986) by William Sears, MD.

>*Addresses the joys and problems of parenthood from the male perspective. Dr. Sears, a pediatrician and father of six, writes from experience. He promises that becoming a father will bring such rich rewards as love, a better marriage, and maturity.*

242 pages/$7.95
Member/$7.15

HYGIEIA: A Woman's Herbal (Freestone Collective Book, 1988) by Jeannine Parvati.

>*Interweaves the ancient practice of herbalism with the new woman's consciousness and holistic health. Covers birth control, menstruation, menopause, pregnancy, childbirth, nursing, psychoactive herbs, abortions, nutritional and self-healing remedies, and infertility.*

247 pages/$13.00
Member/$11.70

Infant Massage: A Handbook for Loving Parents (Bantam Books, 1989) by Vimala Schneider McClure.

>*Sharing and communicating love to your newborn through massage. Helps enhance the bond between you and your infant and gives the father the contact with baby that he often misses. Special chapter on illness and colic. Easy and enjoyable!*

198 pages/$6.95
Member/$6.25

Marie Osmond's Exercises for Mother and Baby (New American Library, 1985) by Elizabeth Noble.

>*An easy-to-use book for shaping up after you've had a baby. Features exercises for you and your baby and tips on postpartum care. Very creative exercises are presented in easy formats. Includes illustrations.*

127 pages/$12.95
Member/$11.65

Positive Pregnancy Fitness: A Guide to a More Comfortable Pregnancy and Easier Birth Through Exercise and Relaxation (Avery Publishing Group, 1988) by Sylvia Klein Olkin.

>*Holistic guide on getting the most out of your pregnancy experience.*
>* *Safe, effective exercises*
>* *Effective stress-management techniques for parents-to-be*
>* *Thorough nutritional information for a healthy mother and baby*
>* *"Inner Bonding"—a new mental technique for connecting the consciousness between mother and baby*
>* *Over 200 illustrations*

254 pages/$9.95
Member/$9.00

Wise Woman Herbal for the Childbearing Year (Ash Tree Publishing Co., 1985) by Susun S. Weed.

>*Comprehensive guide to medicinal herbs that can be used to help relieve many of the stresses of pregnancy and to enhance the labor and birth experience. Well-organized, easy-to-use reference guide.*

171 pages/$8.95
Member/$8.05

AUDIO TAPES-INSTRUCTIONAL

Fundamentals of Yoga I by Sylvia Klein Olkin.
- •Learn techniques to shape and firm your body
- •Learn deep breathing to lower your blood pressure
- •Learn how to totally relax and revitalize
- •FREE illustrated instructional folder included

60 minutes/$11.95
Member/$10.75

Relax and Enjoy: A Stress-Management Program by Sylvia Klein Olkin.
Make relaxation part of your day and enjoy life more!
- •Three separate relaxations included (5-, 10-, and 15-minute relaxations)
- •Accurate directions for releasing tension and fatigue included
- •FREE instructional folder included

40 minutes/$11.95
Member/$10.75

Shape Up!!! by Sylvia Klein Olkin.
Reshape your body, reshape your thinking!
- •Develop a thin self-image
- •Flatten tummy; reduce waist, hips, thighs, and buttocks
- •Eliminate unwanted backaches
- •Tone and strengthen arms/shoulders
- •Illustrated insert card FREE with tape

60 minutes/$11.95
Member/$10.75

Shape Up with Baby by Sylvia Klein Olkin.
Regain your prepregnancy shape (or an even better one!)
- •All directions to the Basic Eight and the Sun and Moon Salutes (Chapter Ten) are found on this tape
- •Flatten tummy; slim hips, thighs, buttocks, and waist
- •Eliminate tension and revitalize body and mind
- •Includes special sing-along exercises just for baby
- •FREE illustrated instructional folder included

60 minutes/$11.95
Member/$10.75

Stress Management by Sylvia Klein Olkin.
Take a few minutes a day to eliminate stress.
- •Contains five special yoga-based stretches designed to eliminate stress from your body
- •Learn proper breathing and meditation to reduce anxieties
- •FREE illustrated instructional folder included

40 minutes/$11.95
Member/$10.75

S-T-R-E-T-C-H-I-N-G for Athletes by Sylvia Klein Olkin.
A limbering alternative to post-athletic-activity aches.
- •Contains directions for seven separate five-minute stretches
- •Includes specific exercises for tight spots
- •FREE illustrated pamphlet included

35 minutes/$11.95
Member/$10.75

S-T-R-E-T-C-H-I-N-G for Runners by Sylvia Klein Olkin.
> *For those who love to run but hate to stretch.*
> • *Contains directions for six separate five-minute stretches*
> • *These effective pre- and post-run stretches will help prevent injuries*
> • *FREE illustrated pamphlet included*

30 minutes/$11.95
Member/$10.75

Fun and Songs and Family Yoga: A Trip Around the World by the Sunflower Yoga Company.
> *Excellent for children of any age. Narrator uses familiar language and favorite songs in combination with easy body movements. Family yoga uses animal images that really attract kids. Is effective in calming kids down, too!*

60 minutes/$11.95
Member/$10.75

AUDIO TAPES-MUSICAL

Adult

Dream Images by Shardad.
> *Guaranteed to put you in a calm, soothing mood via synthesizer and piano music. It is great for tension relief at home or while driving in your car.*

40 minutes/$10.95
Member/$9.85

The Golden Voyage II by Robert Bearns and Ron Dexter.
> *Contains music with a timeless quality that is a blend of natural and environmental sounds, combined with a tapestry of melodic themes. Music is delicately played by classical guitars, flutes, French horns, pianos, string instruments, vibraphones, and synthesizers.*

40 minutes/$10.95
Member/$9.85

I Offer You My Heart by Charley and Lori Thweatt.
> *Charley and Lori are a powerful singing team in their first joint effort. Their original songs include ballads and upbeat pop numbers always with an uplifting message of love and faith. Their joy in singing is contagious and you will feel happier for having listened. Good to use with aerobic workouts.*

40 minutes/$10.95
Member/$9.85

The Living Earth by Annie Locke.
> *Contains scintillating bell-like tones from pianos and synthesizers. Helps ease the listener toward inner peace and relaxation.*

40 minutes/$10.95
Member/$9.85

Miracles by Rob Whitesides-Woo.
> *Combines harp, strings, and winds through sublime melodies calling listeners to journey deep within themselves. A beautiful musical-relaxation tape.*

40 minutes/$10.95
Member/$9.85

Mountain Light by Rob Whitesides-Woo.
> *An exquisite tapestry of instrumental music celebrating the beauty of earth and sky. Exotic flutes, bowed and plucked strings, acoustic and electronic instruments from many lands create a graceful world.*

40 minutes/$10.95
Member/$9.85

Piano Means Soft by Charles Thweatt.
> *Gentle, flowing, peaceful, inner-calming piano music. This tape helps move you to a quiet state of being. The gentle acoustic and electronic piano music helps induce relaxation.*

40 minutes/$10.95
Member $9.85

Piano Whispers by Charles Thweatt.
> *Contains gentle piano music played in a joyous, uplifting manner. Highly recommended to play during baby massage.*

40 minutes/$10.95
Member/$9.85

Sojourn by Scott Fitzgerald and Rob Whitesides-Woo.
> *Contains majestic piano and orchestral music; soothing but uplifting.*

40 minutes/$10.95
Member/$9.85

You Are the Ocean Volumes I and II by Schawkie Roth.
> *Perfect music for relaxation, meditation, or for feeling joyful! Celestial water music is created by blending the sounds of oceans and streams with flute, harp, cello, and zither music. Harmonious melodies interweave.*

Each volume-40 minutes/$10.95
Member/$9.85

Children

Bath Time Magic
> *Turns bath time into fun time as you and your child sing along. Features contemporary and traditional water-play songs. Lyrics enclosed. (Ages 1-10)*

40 minutes/$10.95
Member/$9.85

Happiness Cake by Linda Arnold.
> *Another award-winning tape by Linda featuring old favorites like "Puff the Magic Dragon" and "Be a Friend." The new songs, such as "Happiness Cake" and "There's a Dinosaur Knocking at My Door," are imaginative and delightful. (Ages 2-10)*

40 minutes/$10.95
Member/$9.85

Lullaby Magic
> *Ease your child into peaceful sleep at quiet time or bedtime with soothing lullabies from Brahms to the Beatles. These beautiful lullabies appeal to children and parents as well. (Ages birth-5)*

40 minutes/$10.95
Member/$9.85

Lullaby Magic II
Discover those intimate moments with your children as you lull them to sleep with well-known favorites by such artists as Elvis Presley, Judy Garland, and the Mamas and the Papas. (Ages birth-5)

40 minutes/$10.95
Member/$9.85

Make Believe by Linda Arnold.
Imagination is your key as you fly to a land of fantasy where balloons become moons, vegetables sing, and dinosaurs go sailing by. With charming simplicity in a variety of styles, Linda's joyous songs will delight the entire family. Contains twenty-one songs. (Ages 2-10)

40 minutes/$10.95
Member/$9.85

Morning Magic
1987 Parent's Choice Honor Award winner. Feature contemporary and traditional wake-up songs written by such artists as the Beatles, James Taylor, and Paul Simon. A perfect way to start the day, end a nap, or use during play time. (Ages 1-6)

40 minutes/$10.95
Member/$9.85

Play, Sing and Dream by Carroll Mailhot.
Features a beautiful, creative collection of songs to sing along with or to dream by. Side 1 includes active play songs; side 2 features lullabies. Carroll sings along with her own children, combining her expertise as an actress with a clear soprano voice to create an enchanting tape. (Ages 2-10)

40 minutes/$10.95
Member/$9.85

Sillytime Magic
1989 Parent's Choice Award winner. Brighten your child's play time with silly songs. Get into the magic of childhood with this fun tape. (Ages 2-10)

40 minutes/$10.95
Member/$9.85

Teaching Peace by Red Grammer.
Teaching Peace is addictive and fun to play over and over again! A wonderful tape for teaching children values and for learning how to cope with disturbing things in their lives. Red sings with kids in the recording studio. His joy in singing songs that he and his wife wrote shines through on this magical tape. (Ages 2-10)

40 minutes/$10.95
Member/$9.85

Travelin' Magic
Turn any trip, whether real or make-believe, into a sing-along party. Terrific travelin' tunes about cars, buses, trains, and planes. (Ages 2-10)

40 minutes/$10.95
Member/$9.85

Babies

Baby Go To Sleep
This special tape can induce your newborn to sleep at an appropriate time. Contains classic lullabies sung in combination with

the sound of a human heartbeat. Actually calms and causes sleep in nine out of every ten infants tested. Why tolerate a fussy baby? Get the Baby Go To Sleep tape because it really works! Also works for pre-school children.

35 minutes/$12.95
Member/$11.75

Lullabies from Around the World by Steven Bergman.
Gentle lullabies from around the world. Calming for mothers, babies, and children of all ages. Also helpful in reducing stress.

40 minutes/$10.95
Member/$9.85

Slumberland by Steven Bergman.
Flutes, guitars, strings, and synthesizers are combined with birds, crickets, and heartbeats to help create a calming environment for baby.

40 minutes/$10.95
Member/$9.85

Sweet Baby Dreams by Steven Bergman.
Lullaby music includes the gentle sound of a heartbeat. Great for relaxing and quieting newborns as well as young children and expectant mothers.

40 minutes/$10.95
Members/$9.85

VIDEO TAPES

Baby Joy: Exercise and Activities for Parents and Infants by Elizabeth Noble, PT, and Leo Sorger, MD.

Foster a love of music and movement in your baby as you speed your postpartum recovery with exercises that you can do alone, with your baby, and with your spouse. Join Elizabeth and Leo with their son Carsten for a fun-filled hour of joy. Features postpartum and post-Cesarean section exercises, ball and trampoline aerobics and stretches, activities for parent-infant pairs, baby movement and massage, water games, and infant stimulation. Fun and educational!

60 minutes VHS/$45.00
Member/$40.50

Positive Parenting Fitness Exercise Routines for Mommy and Baby by Liz Schneider.
Liz exercises with her class using many of the exercises found in Chapter Thirteen. Has perky music, excellent techniques, and important cautions. (Available after June, 1992).

60 minutes VHS/$29.95
Member/$26.00

Infant Massage: An Instructional Video by Cheryl Brenman Productions.
This video contains a step-by-step lesson on how to give a practical and enjoyable massage for the infant as well as the older child. Infant massage helps you nourish your baby emotionally; teaches relaxation skills; stimulates respiratory, circulatory, and gastrointestinal functions in your child; and helps build confidence in your parenting skills. Friendly, easy manner used throughout this educational film. For a better beginning, massage your infant!

60 minutes VHS/$39.95
Member/$36.00

Your Baby: A Video Guide to Care and Understanding with Penelope Leach.

This film provides a comprehensive and practical guide for newborn care and development. Penelope Leach, noted child-development expert and best-selling author of Your Baby and Child, demonstrates techniques of everyday care and teaches exactly what your baby needs from you in a variety of situations. Topics include meeting your baby, bringing baby home, feeding the baby, how to comfort a crying baby, etc. Each topic is presented in a separate section and is color coded for easy preview.

77 minutes VHS/$29.95
Member/$26.00

PARENTING PRODUCTS

Almond Glow Skin Lotion
Calming massage oil. An Edgar Cayce formulation. Use as massage oil, suntan oil, or bath oil. Can be used for nipple preparation before breastfeeding. Helps relieve the discomfort of stretch marks. Contains all-natural ingredients: pure peanut oil, virgin olive oil, lanolin oil, almond oil, and Vitamin E. Available in the following scents: light flourishing almond, coconut musk, and jasmine.

2 ounces/$2.00   8 ounces/$6.50
Member/$1.85   Member/$5.85

Indicate desired scent (almond, coconut musk, jasmine, or uncented)

Lanolin for Nursing Mothers
Made of 100 percent pure anhydrous lanolin, this is an exceptionally fine product for conditioning the breastfeeding mother's tender nipples.

1.3 ounces/$3.95
Member/$3.50

Free and Dry Breast-Care Shields
Feather-light, flesh-colored shields worn over breasts inside the bra to collect and contain milk leakage. Helps eliminate stains due to leakage, helps correct inverted nipples, and helps relieve cracked nipples. Comes with its own carrying case.

Pair/$7.00
Member/$6.30

Happy Family Breast Pump
A pain-free, totally effective breast pump that helps breastfeeding mothers express milk for later feedings; also relieves engorged breasts. Constructed of non-breakable, dishwasher-safe plastic, this American-made pump features two sizes of breast cups. Converts into a bottle with an orthodontic nipple.

Manual pump/$25.00
Member/$22.50

Battery-Operated Breast Pump
Takes all the work out of pumping your breasts—saves time, too. This unit comes complete with batteries, collection bottle, vacuum chamber, pump, bottle top and cap, nipple, and instructions printed in three languages. Features suction control and suction-release button. Very easy to operate.

Battery-operated pump/$39.50
Member/$35.50

Dyna-Band

Dyna-Bands are thin strips of latex (six inches wide by three feet long) that come in light- and medium-weight resistance. During exercise, they provide outside resistance for your muscles.Dyna Band exercises are safe for strength training during pregnancy and after.

Each Dyna-Band is imprinted with the Positive Pregnancy and Parenting Logo. Also available is a complete guide for strength training, which includes rules and tips for strength training, proper body alignment, and suggested music to train by.

Dyna-Band/$5.00   With Guide/$9.95
Member/$4.50   Member/$9.00

Indicate desired resistance (light or medium) when ordering.

Light-Weight Exercise Mat

This extremely light-weight (ten ounces), non-slippable, 19x72 inch exercise mat comes with closeable straps and a plastic carrying case. Available in mint green or powder blue.

Exercise mat/$10.95
Member/$10.00

Indicate desired color (mint green or powder blue) when ordering.

Positive Pregnancy and Parenting Fitness Maternity or Postpartum T-Shirt

Great for exercising in or for just lounging around in, this 100 percent cotton T-shirt comes with the Positive Pregnancy and Parenting Fitness logo imprinted across the front. Washing instructions included. Something every woman should own and enjoy!

L & XL /$14.00   XXL /$14.00
Member/$12.60   Member/$12.60
(pink)   (white)

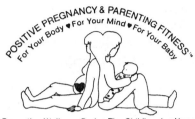

Promoting Wellness During The Childbearing Years

Red Raspberry Leaf Tea

The most recommended tea for pregnancy, childbirth, and the postpartum period. Helps eliminate nausea, prepares the uterus for labor and birth, and helps the postpartum body to heal. This best-known herbal aid also includes "The Red Raspberry Leaf Story."

1 ounce/$1.25   2 ounces/$2.25
Member/$1.00   Member/$2.00

5 ounces/$4.50
Member/$4.00

Red Raspberry Leaf Tea in Capsule Form

This herbal tonic for pregnancy, childbirth, and the postpartum period is now available in 400 mg. capsules. Simply open one capsule and sprinkle the contents into one cup of boiling water, stir, and enjoy your instant red raspberry tea! Can be taken in capsule form, too. A "no-fuss" way to enjoy this tea all through pregnancy and postpartum. Each safety-sealed bottle contains 100 capsules. Also included is "The Red Raspberry Leaf Story."

100 capsules/$8.00
Member/$7.20

Jolly Jumper Natural Baby Food Mill

Be assured your baby is getting nutrition with no additives! Save money, too. This hand-operated food mill has a spoon-out spout. Great for outings! Made of high-impact plastic that is dishwasher safe, this food mill is easily disassembled for cleaning.

One/$8.00   Two/$15.00
Member/$7.20   Member/$13.50

Happy Baby Carrier

Help soothe and relieve your baby's anxiety when he encounters new people and places. When you carry your baby up front, he can either face you or the world! Features: snap-off infant head support, front- or back-carrying capacity, double-strength seat, leg room that grows with baby, and padded straps and leg openings. Perfect comfort and safety. Available in red (solid fabric) or blue (mesh—a summertime favorite). Polyester, completely washable.

Carrier/$19.95
Member/$18.00

Indicate color (red-solid fabric or blue-mesh) when ordering.

Pregnant women and new mothers should always check with their health care providers before taking any herbs.

Resources for New Parents

ORGANIZATIONS

American Academy of Pediatrics (AAP)
141 Northwest Point Boulevard
PO Box 927
Elk Grove Village, IL 60009-0927

AAP has an extensive catalog of publications including inexpensive pamphlets on such topics as first-aid and child-restraint systems.

American College of Nurse Midwives
(ACNM)
1522 K Street NW, Suite 1000
Washington, DC 20005
(202) 289-0171
FAX (202) 289-4395

ACNM establishes and maintains standards for the practice of certified nurse-midwives. Call for referral of nurse-midwives in your area.

American College of Obstetrics
and Gynecologists (ACOG)
Resource Center
409 Twelfth Street SW

Washington, DC 20024
(202) 638-5577

ACOG sets national standards in obstetrical education and practice. A wide variety of free patient-information booklets are available upon request.

American Foundation for Maternal
and Child Health
30 Beekman Place
New York, NY 10022
(212) 759-5510

This foundation acts as a clearinghouse on birth and postpartum practices. Pamphlets available.

Cesarean Prevention Movement (CPM)
PO Box 152
Syracuse, NY 13210
(315) 424-1942

CPM is dedicated to lowering unnecessary Cesarean deliveries, which occur at an alarmingly high rate in the United States. It encourages vaginal birth after a Cesarean. CPM sponsors classes on how to avoid a Cesarean delivery.

317

Write or call for further information. Newsletter available.

Childhelp, USA
The National Child-Abuse Hotline
24 hours—7 days a week
(800) 4-A-CHILD
(800) 422-4453

Confidential listeners help harried mothers. Sometimes you need someone who is calm and objective to listen to you.

The Children's Foundation
725 15th Street NW
Suite 505
Washington, DC 20005
(202) 347-3300

Provides information on food programs such as the Women's, Infants and Children (WIC) program.

Compassionate Friends
PO Box 3696
Oak Brook, IL 60522-3696
(708) 990-0010

Provides support and encouragement for parents who have lost a child. Chapters throughout the world. Call for local referral.

COPE
530 Tremont Street
Boston, MA 02116
(617) 357-5588

COPE (Coping with the Overall Pregnancy/ Parenting Experience) provides telephone support. Also offers information on national support groups for parents.

Depression After Delivery
PO Box 1282
Morrisville, PA 19067
(215) 295-3994

Counseling over the phone for depressed mothers. Call and talk to someone who can really help. Network throughout the country. Call for local chapter.

International Childbirth Education Association (ICEA)
PO Box 20048
Minneapolis, MN 55420
(612) 854-8660
(800)624-4934

ICEA is a non-profit organization that unites people who support family-centered maternity care; they believe in freedom of choice based on knowledge of alternatives of mother and newborn. Operates a mail-order bookstore.

International Association of Infant Massage Instructors
PO Box 16103
Portland, OR 97216
(503) 253-9977

Provides resources (instructions, oils, books, videos, etc.) for parents and professionals on the subject of infant massage.

La Leche League International (LLLI)
PO Box 1209
9616 Minneapolis Avenue
Franklin Park, IL 60131
(708) 451-1891
(800) LA LECHE

LLLI is an international breastfeeding support group for new mothers. There are local chapters throughout the United States. A newsletter, mail-order catalog, and other literature is available for non-members.

National Foundation of the March of Dimes
1275 Mamaroneck Avenue
White Plains, NY 10605
(914) 428-7100

The March of Dimes distributes free pamphlets and fact sheets on pregnancy and postpartum. Catalog available.

National Health Information Clearinghouse
PO Box 1133
Washington, DC 20013
(800) 336-4797

A source of information for any health-related problem of both children and adults.

Parents Anonymous
6733 South Sepulveda Boulevard
Suite 270
Los Angeles, CA 90045
(800) 421-0353

Telephone, crisis-intervention support group for parents who abuse or who are afraid that they might abuse their child. Call national number for a local referral.

Perinatal Health and Fitness Network
PO Box 3092
Stony Creek, CT 06405

National Organization to create a professional identity and standards of practice, and to provide information about training and certifica-

tion for pregnancy and parenting fitness educators. Write for classes and membership information. Send $1.00 and self-addressed business-sized envelope for information and latest newsletter.

Positive Pregnancy and Parenting Fitness
51 Saltrock Road
Baltic, CT 06330
(800) 433-5523
(203) 822-8573

Trains and certifies pregnancy and parenting fitness teachers throughout the United States. Has newsletter, books, audio and video tapes, and other pregnancy and parenting information. Send $1.00 along with your name and address for a copy of the most recent newsletter.

BOOKSTORES

Birth and Life Bookstore
7001 Alonzo Avenue NW
Seattle, WA 98107
(800) 736-0631
(206) 789-4444

A mail-order bookstore specializing in pregnancy, postpartum, and child raising. Hundreds of titles available, many that are out of print. Call for free catalog.

Informed Birth and Parenting Bookstore
501 Berkley Avenue
Ann Arbor, MI 48103
(313) 662-6857

This mail-order bookstore specializes in publication for those planning home births. Pregnancy and postpartum books and information are also available.

MAGAZINES

Twins
PO Box 12045
Overland Park, KS 66212
(800) 821-5533
(313) 722-1090

International magazine for parents of twins or multiples. Twins features families of multiples and research on this subject.

American Baby
475 Park Avenue South
New York, NY 10016
(212) 689-3600

Call or write for a free sample copy.

The Compleat Mother Magazine
Box 209
Minot, ND 58702
(701) 852-2822

Call or write for a free sample copy.

MANUFACTURERS

Equinox Botanicals
Route 1 Box 71
Rutland, OH 45775
(614) 742-2581

Makers of high-quality herbal salves and tinctures for pregnancy and postpartum. Free catalog.

Herb-Pharm
PO Box 116
Williams, OR 97544
(503) 846-7178

Recognized as an innovative leader in the American herb industry, Herb-Pharm was founded and directed twelve years ago by "Herbal Ed" Smith. All herbs sold by this company are cultivated without the use of chemical fertilizers, pesticides, or herbicides. They are hand-harvested, shade-dried, and then promptly formulated while still fresh and succulent. Herbs are never fumigated or irradiated. Free illustrated catalog available.

Liberty Products
PO Box 66068
Portland, OR 97266
(800) 289-8427

Features quality massage and bath oils, natural baby teething oil, and other natural baby products. Wholesale only.

Mountain Spirit
PO Box 368
Port Townsend, WA 98368
(206) 385-4491

This family-owned mail-order business carries a complete line of herbal supplies ranging from tinctures and teas to a full line of birthing supplies and medicinal products. With a strong focus on young children and new mothers, Mountain Spirit uses only organically grown or wildcrafted herbs in their extensive variety of products. Only the finest cold-pressed oils are used and everything is prepared by hand. Send $1.00 for current 24-page catalog.

About the Author

Sylvia Klein Olkin has a Masters degree in Education/Eastern Studies. She is currently the director of Positive Pregnancy and Parenting Fitness, an organization that has trained and certified over 650 instructors in the United States, Canada, and England to teach holistic fitness programs. She is the author of *Positive Pregnancy Through Yoga* and *Positive Pregnancy Fitness.* Ms. Olkin is an international speaker on all aspects of yoga and pregnancy/parenting fitness. She has appeared on numerous radio and television talk shows and has had a number of magazine articles published. She is a member of the Board of Advisors of the Pre and Perinatal Psychology Association, the Perinatal Health and Fitness Network, and the National Association of Childbirth Assistants. She lives in Connecticut with her husband and two sons.

Index

Blues. *See* Postpartum blues.
Bodily elimination, 36
Borage tea, 41
Braun, Maureen, RN, BN, 128
Breast infection (mastitis), 37. *See also*
    Engorged or painful breasts.
Breast pumps, 95
Breast shields, 96
Breastfeeding, 89-97
    and La Leche League, 96
    and sex, 93
    attitudes toward, 94-95
    basic information on, 89-90
    cautions and comments on, 96-97
    correct positioning for, 92
    equipment for, 95-96
    physical aspects of, 92
Breathing, controlled, 14-16
    calming, 17-20
    physiology of, 15-16
    rejuvenating, 20-22
Brewer, Gail, 63
Bridge, The, 132
Burkhardt, Grace, RN, 265
Burzycki, Jacquie, 63
Butterfly Stretch, 171
Buttocks Slimmer, 201

Caffeine, 73
Calcium, as part of balanced diet, 64-65
    daily serving suggestions, 66
Calcium-Rich Tea recipe, 79-80
Calendula, 33
Calf/Thigh/Hip Toner, 233
Calories,luxury, 71, 72
Camomile, 30
Carbohydrates, as part of balanced diet, 65
    daily serving suggestions, 67-68
Catnip tea, 45
Cervical cap, 112
Cesarean delivery, 127-133
    comfort measures, 127-128
    exercises after, 129-133
Cesarean-section complaints, 32-34
Charging Breath, 21
Chest Expander, 251
Chest Presses, 202

Cleansing Breath, 20
Clogged milk ducts, 38, 90
Cobra, The, 246
Coleman, Libby, 111
Comfort, Alex, PhD, 111
Comfrey compress, 30, 31, 33, 38, 40
Condoms, 112
Constipation. *See* Bodily elimination.
**Constructive Relaxation Breathing (Your
    Mini-Vacation),** 19
Contraceptive implants, 112
Contraceptives. *See* Birth control.
Contractions. *See* After pains.
Cool-down period, proper, 184
Cowlin, Ann, MA, 115
Crib Squats, 258
Crying and postpartum blues, 53
Curl-Backs with Baby, 216
Cystitis, 36

Daily routine and exercise, 253-258
Daisy leaf compress, 38
Depression, 41. *See also* Postpartum blues;
    Postpartum depression.
Diaphragm, 112
Diet
    and ideal weight, 59-60
    and nursing mother, 51-52, 60, 61
    and postpartum blues, 50-51
    and postpartum weight loss, 60-61
    See also Safe Reducing Diet; Weight-loss
    programs.
D.I.E.T. for Pregnancy, 76
Dyna-Bands
    cautions, 186
    how to use, 187-188
    rules and tips, 188

Elevator, The, 103
Elimination. *See* Bodily elimination.
Endorphins, 42
Energizing Single-Nostril Breath, 22
Engorged or painful breasts, 39
Erick, Miriam, 76
Estrogen levels, 93, 99
Exercise. *See* Aerobics, low-impact; Baby
    movement program; Backaches,